Eat Right Now

The End of Mindless Eating
Vegetarian / Vegan / Raw Recipes
Food Essays

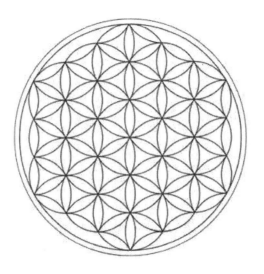

Chef Wendell Fowler

www.chefwendell.com

Self-help requires intelligence, common sense, mindfulness and compassion, love of self, and accountability for your actions. The information in this book is offered with the desire to empower humanity to take a greater responsibility for their health destiny. Always seek the advice of a licensed Integrative Holistic MD.

To order single or bulk copies of the book, or to arrange for Chef Wendell Fowler to enlighten your social group or corporate employees, contact:

chefwendellfowler@gmail.com
twitter.com/wendellfowler
www.facebook.com/wendell.fowler.16

317-372-2592

First Printing:
©2013 by Wendell R. Fowler.

Second Printing:
©2014 by Wendell R. Fowler

Edited by: Zach 'Artie' Dunkin
Cover design by Malarie Piercy

4

To Sandi

My Angel Eyes

Crystal Love and Kisses

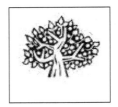

Essay Index

Recipe Index

Zesty Dragon Bowl 195

Soups

Red Lentil Soup w/Coconut & Curry 196
Chilled Corn Bisque w/Curry Oil 197
Winter Vegetable Stew 198
Green Chili Tortilla Soup 198
Vegan Mushroom Soup 199
Lima Bean Soup 199

Salads, Vegetables, Sides & Fruits

Spinach Salad w/Beets & Oranges 200
Polynesian Coconut Bowl 200
Broccoli & Tempeh "Anti-Cancer"
  Salad with Peanut Dressing ® 201
Crispy Crunch Summer Salad 202
Quinoa Walnut Cherry Salad 202
Asian Quinoa with Summer Vegetables 203
Mediterranean Quinoa Salad 204
Jicama-Orange Salad w/Summer Berries 205
Hoosier Tomato, Basil & Corn Salad 206
Avocado on the Half-shell: the Alligator
  Pear 206
Spicy Thai Style Slaw 207
Sweet and Sour Kale Salad 207
Sicilian Garden Salad 218
Kale and Grapefruit Salad 209
Spicy Orange Slaw 209
Dairy Free Ranch Dressing
  via My Whole Food Life 209
Sweet Curry Dressing w/Tahini 210
Coconut Mayonnaise 210
Vodka Spiked Cherry Tomatoes
  with Pepper and Salt 211
Tomato Quinoa Risotto 211
Vegan Tempeh Potato Patties 212
Tangy Marinated Vegetables 212
Green Beans, Potatoes and Spinach
  in Coconut Curry 213
Seared Green Beans w/Garlic & Chiles 214
Yellow Basmati Rice 214
Cilantro Lime Rice 215

Desserts and Goodies

Beverages

Awards and Kudos

- Host / Contributor WISH TV 8 Weekend Daybreak News in Indianapolis since 2003.
- 2005, 2006, 2007, 2009 Gold and Silver Medals, North America Mature Publishers Association (NAMPA): *Indianapolis Prime Times* column
- 2004, Bronze Medal, The National Mature Media: *Indianapolis Prime Times* column 2002, Silver Medal, Magazine/Newspaper Article Series, NAMPA: *Indianapolis Prime Times* column
- 2002, Merit Award, National Media Awards (in competition with national publications such as *Modern Maturity and Prevention Magazine): Indianapolis Prime Times* column
- 2001, Gold Medal, NAMPA: *Indianapolis Prime Times* column
- 2001, Silver Medal, NAMPA: *Indianapolis Prime Times* column
- 1993 and 1992, Bronze Medals, The American Culinary Association Invitation Competition, Indianapolis, Indiana

Introduction

I no longer fear death, and have no ambitions of living 100 earth years. My goal is to feel good, to be kind and to become the best I was created to be...*now*; today and not later; to vibrate at my highest social, spiritual, cosmic, and career level by caring compassionately for my Holy Temple with food, exercise, acts of kindness, self-love, and quiet meditation: loving myself so much that I no longer want to make myself needlessly suffer.

How can your 'greater good' ever find you if you're buried beneath the festering rabble of the low-grade nutrition disgorged upon a trusting society by Big Food, bankers and agribusiness?

The vast majority of Americans believe it's possible to have a great deal of control over their level of physical activity, the healthfulness of their diet, and their weight, yet far fewer are actually taking control. Disease is born from the lack of nutritional insight; malnutrition. Since the start of the Industrial Revolution's 100 year lie, we've been intentionally betrayed by the food industry and led to perceive food as convenient entertainment rather than heavenly cellular nutrition. When you see the true nature of your suffering and disease, you are liberated.

21st Century disconnected Americans eat more than any other nation. Yet, testing the over-fed and under-exercised obese reveal they're malnourished; operating on a damaged system. Experts say the pigswill composing the addictive American diet of fat, salt, sugar, white flour, caffeine, tobacco and alcohol with insanely high sugar calories, but low on authentic human nutrition, is the keystone of preventable disease in the land o' plenty. Until I was forty, lingering on my ICU death bed, I, too, had eaten poorly. But the Grim Reaper dropped by to poke me. I acknowledged my vegaphobic diet of KFC, doughnuts, bacon burgers, Mt. Dew, Jerky, booze and sugary foods nearly killed me. I didn't love myself sufficiently. Self-love is the highest form of affection. Your Temple is the vehicle for your spirit and your soul. It is the piece of the universe you've been assigned to tend and cherish. I am love. I am joy. I am freedom. I am peace.

I am peaceful, whole, and balanced, but only if I feed my cells what they require to thrive.

The disease of obesity is the new malnutrition. Obesity from empty calories sets in, and your brain stops growing, rendering you less than whole. Disease is most frequently caused by a nutritional deficiency. Vitamins, minerals and enzymes are building blocks your cells need to sustain whole health. Logically without 40 basic vitamins and 90 trace minerals needed daily, your trillions of cells cannot sustain a crumbling Temple. Eating healthy foods is compassionate self-love. If your spiritual antennae are 'funkied' up from eating dead food, then how can you connect effectively with the infinite river of the Cosmos boundless energy and intelligence?

When I cradle a bowl of the cosmos's bounty, I vibrate with gratitude. Forty thousand children die every day because of the lack of food and there's a famine in Africa. You don't need to be in a monastery to practice this, but practice self-love; the most sincere love for oneself. Eating mindfully and gratefully at your dinner table is a wonderful way to nourish compassion.

Our Holy Temples are sacred. Mindful eating embodies a peaceful message of re-connecting to earth, supporting sustainable growing practices and empowering people to heal with food and herbs. Exactly what our world needs in these toxic times; not more separation, adversity and competition. We cannot be compassionate to others until we are first compassionate with ourselves. Without compassion, the world will continually war, my friends. Compassionate, mindful consumption will eventually save us.

Come together...right now. Co-create a joy filled world that nourishes mind, the 7 Major Chakras and our spiritual energy. Eating a plant-based diet will make you more compassionate, connected, calm and loving. Compassionate eating gives us opportunity to actualize a humane and peaceful lifestyle honoring all sentient beings who share life on this earthly plane. Behaviors should be consistent with our values. Eating empathetically will shift civilization's consciousness. Compassionate consumption breeds non-violence, kindness and love for all beings. We are all intimately connected.

Eat Right Now is a combination of a plant-based, peace-filled diet, provocative food essays, scandalous information regarding America's toxic, corrupt food system and a vegan / vegetarian / raw cookbook promoting and supporting the family farm and the local artisan community who lovingly grow and craft living foods and goods. It is designed with the intention of reducing nutritional illiteracy in America; dietary self-defense from the onslaught of nutritionally bankrupt processed foods passed off by miscreant "corporate America" monsters as wholesome and nutritious, when indeed, their inferior twaddle nurtures heartbreaking, costly disease. Americans living in the greatest country on this blue-green planet are malnourished. So, what is terrorism? Who should we fear most, our government for allowing toxic foods into the food supply, Monsanto, Chem-trails, Con Agra, lilting food mascots, mentally damaged food corporation creatures in need of love, or the innate malleability of suggestible Americans unaware of closed door, boardroom, and Fat Cat, Good-Ole-Boy chicanery going on behind a patriotic country's trusting backs? We're on our own, fellow stardust.

Like sleeping and breathing, the quality and authenticity of what we eat is infinitely more important for the species' survival than anyone has been led to believe. People not only expect food to taste good, but now they look to food to address specific health problems. However, narcissistic Americans are more concerned about their physical appearance, social status, politics, what car they drive, and their empty material possessions than their Temple's essentials. How can America defend itself from proliferating pandemics of largely avoidable diseases and obesity if they've not experienced the joyous feel-good results of eating fresh, local and pure? The bungled and biased Standard American Diet (SAD) oozes across the crusty kitchen floor, seething with artificial toxic chemicals, food colorings, carbon monoxide, MSG, Round-Up, pesticides, antibiotics, hormones, and constellations of ungodly amalgams not meant to enter the sacrosanct Holy Temple, our only true home.

The best kept secret in mainstream medicine is that under the right conditions, your body can heal itself. Civilization's greatest human tragedy is the ill-fated priority of chemical therapy over fresh, living nutrition, the substitution of artificial therapy over natural, of poisons over nourishment. Food, not considered medicinal by most, has become the taproot of social entertainment, instant gratification and pleasure, social status, comfort, tradition, convenience, and a means to profit. We've failed to place food in context with disease, especially significant when the body isn't receiving the right tools or nutrients to repair injured or damaged cells. Like rebuilding a rickety aging home, quality materials are central to the outcome. Nourishment by food is the process by which your Holy Temple assimilates and digests food, then uses it for mental, spiritual, and physical growth, healing, and tissue replacement. The dilemma is, for many decades, we've been hard-wired by smart bomb advertising and disinformation to love, accept and consume dead industrial-strength faux food. Ergo wholesome foods have become an acquired taste. Once again, quite bluntly, America, the greatest country on this beautiful blue earth, is suffering malnutrition. Wendell Berry put it succinctly: "People are fed by the food industry which pays no attention to health, and we are treated by the health industry, which pays no attention to food."

In this enjoyable read, I jubilantly share results the ethereal Universal Apothecary has on mind, body, and "soulular" connectivity and that the low-grade Western Diet seasoned with deceit, plastic food, chemicals, hormones, and a piquant stew of crappy compounds was not destined by our Creator to be ingested. Our God did not lovingly create us to be sickly. Each short attention span food essay contains "hot off the griddle" scientific food information, philosophy, encouragement, history, hunting and foraging tips, resources, and heaps of love seasoned with healthy cynicism.

Despite boasting the best, albeit most costly healthcare on earth, the U.S. is the 49th unhealthiest nation. Healthcare and illiterate SAD standards have failed miserably; prevention is shunned, greed and gluttony are idolized. Consequently, a great nation suffers pointlessly. Chef Wendell will reboot your food perceptions and help connect the dots between largely preventable chronic disease and the current diet we dearly worship.

The contemporary zeitgeist we see in the proliferation of chronic disease, obesity, depression, and the growing population of aggressive, greedy bullies, is the result of the same thing: dietary imbalances in the seven underlying key systems in your Holy Temple; the foundation of health, mental acuity, spiritual connectivity, happiness and disease. Sadly, one cannot connect effectively with their higher source or meet their glorious potential when malnourished from the SAD of altered, machine cuisine; *greedy, soulless bullies in need of love*.

Earthlings not only expect food to taste good but now they wisely look to food to address preventable health problems. Paradoxically, healthy, living, fresh food has become an acquired taste. Messed up, eh? Through years of indulgence and corporate bastardization of wholesome living food for profit, not the greater good, many have become addicted hostage to a perverted appetite, literally addicted to low-grade food. There's no time like 'the now' to welcome wholesome, local living foods into your daily menu. In my many talks, I encourage audiences, "It's never too late to let go of self- destructive eating behaviors and re-learn how to eat all over again and discover the joy and bliss resulting from eating what our cells crave." Once you're aware of the many, many unholy chemicals lurking in your food and what's they are monstrously doing to your heath, you'll be prepared to make better food decisions which will help you and your families rise above self-destructive eating behaviors, preventing everyone from achieving their inborn potential. Peace, love, joy and light to each soul who reads and notes these compassion-seasoned words. It's entirely up to you; we're all on our own in this vast sea of gloopy food flotsam. You are so worthy, beautiful; your family needs and loves you, so return that love by cooking real food that will transcend them into their cosmic greatness.

1
Food and Spirituality: My Journey to Mindfulness

Hosting a CBS TV Healthy Eating segment since 2004 put me in position to witness the glorious outcomes of eating a healthy, plant-based, non-violent diet of real food, not crappy machine cuisine. It's true you can lead the proverbial horse to water and occasionally you meet a grateful horse. Nutritional illiteracy in America is a costly, preventable epidemic. The best kept hidden secret in mainstream corporate medicine is, under the right conditions, your Temple can heal itself.

Kind folks share they've applied this food literacy activists' dietary advice to their meal plan and daily lifestyle with joyful results. It's not rocket science. On my advice, a gentleman wisely decided to quit drinking diet beverages and his triglycerides plunged to normal for the first time in decades. Another middle-aged weekend warrior said eating healthier enabled him to recapture the energy and vitality of a 25 year old. A lovely senior gal ecstatically shared her mental acuity had improved so much she had more self-esteem and optimism. They all agree it wasn't easy breaking life-long, hard-wired eating habits, but with resolve, it wasn't long till their lives rotated 180 degrees for the better. They all mentioned they were much more centered and grounded.

The most inspiring result of re-educating folks to feed their Holy Temple according to our Creator's bill of fare came after one of my performances. I totally relate. One particular gal's eyes shimmered with what I perceived as tears of sadness. She fully hugged me and began: "I'm happier; more at peace. I've developed a better connection with my Creator and feel closer to Him. My family says I'm no longer a grouchy bitch. The kids tell me they actually like me and hug me and tell me they love me more often. My husband says I'm easier to get along with." Queue goose bumps of joy. I recognized her tears sprung from joy, not sorrow.

After shaking the Grim Reaper's skeletal hand 23 years ago, overcoming viral heart disease, KFC, Krispy Kremes, obesity, and sloth, I received the cosmos' life mission for me, re-educate the masses. The Great Creator hit this clueless ADD writer with a cosmic 2 X 4 to get my attention. When I stopped eating dead, fake food, I gradually reconnected with, and became closer to the Divine. With restored body, mind, intention and enhanced heavenly lines of communication, I discovered who I truly was. Adhering to God's dietary maintenance plan, I too began connecting clearer with the Great Spirit.

Willingly adopting a non-violent plant food diet gave my Temple loftier reception to the gentle whispers of a loving Creator. I became a satellite dish on steroids.

When earthlings deeply nourish their Holy Temple's trillions of cells, they'll vibrate in blissful harmony, opening crystal clear lines of communication to our expanding universe and become more intimate with their higher source. When dead junk food is the sources of fuel, symbolic pipes get clogged, wiring frayed and plugs misfire, hence we're less than our potential and celestial communication becomes garbled.

There are some who will never change no matter what. We get it love you unconditionally. However, more folks are joyously awakening and steward their Holy Temple. One fact is true, it's not your fault. You've been aggressively encouraged to depart the road of nutritional righteousness because it's obscenely profitable. Science can land a satellite on Saturn but won't spend a dime communicating unbiased eating behaviors that advance and perpetuate the species for the greater good of all. You are infinitely more powerful than you've been led to believe.

My passage into veganism was akin to unpeeling layers of knowledge and the unfolding of self. The non-violent lifestyle led me to discover more about myself and the glorious world where I live even as it whispered clues my soul has always known.

After nearly taking an eternal nap on the wrong side of the sod due to terminal viral heart disease, I evolved from an all-you-can-eat carnivore to vegetarian to a 90% vegan with rawist tendencies, something incomprehensible considering I ate meat three times daily for 40 years. When I gave up meat over 23 years ago, people asked me why. When I said I cared too much about the animals, I'd get a lot of eyes rolling back in people's heads. Once I started explaining it was for health reasons, people kept quiet, knowing deep down inside it isn't healthy to eat today's conventional, carbon monoxide-preserved meat. Science recently supported this finding.

After all, even the purest vegetarian, raw or vegan diet is primarily concerned with the body which is temporary and about to wither and die. Mahatma Gandhi made it clear when he wrote, "The vegetarian diet is for the building of the spirit and not of the body. Man is more than meat. It is this spirit in us for which we are concerned." Illogically, we currently live in a society where people are fed by Big Food which pays absolutely no attention to human health, and we are treated by the health care industry which pays absolutely no attention to the healing majesty of real, living, locally sourced food. Irresponsible behavior fed by the offensive disease of greed.

Are food, health, and longevity important to man or is spiritual understanding the ultimate goal in life? I learned our Holy Temple responds positively to a vegetarian diet and can help us achieve the highest vibration. Awakened earthlings are moving towards non-violent veganism in droves. They're discovering that the connection between food, spirituality, and 'soulular' growth is far deeper than man is able to imagine. We are merely molecules perceived as matter; the universe experiencing itself in human form. No one is the material body, but each of us is an eternal, individual, spirit soul inhabiting a particular body—loving servants to the Great Creator. I kept asking myself, "Do I not have the responsibility to live my life for the highest purpose?"

My left brain spends hours researching the physical impact that consumption of today's meat and dairy has on animals, civilization, human health, air and water quality, purity, and availability, and ultimately, planet earth in general. After years of research, my brain has become an archive of hot-off-the-griddle scientific statistics, quotes, food history and facts. Knowledge supports and centers me in challenging debate with those who question my sanity. It also exhilarates those wishing to cross over to the green side. Most green newbies learn quickly veganism is a destination, not the starting point.

The spiritual side of veganism is harder to define. How do you tell skeptics "my spirit engages in a joyful dance as I shop community farmers markets or allow my hands to work with whole grains, seeds, and sun-drenched green garden produce and then turn everything into delightful family nourishment?" When you are eating live foods, you're getting the vibrating life force from our mutual, living planet. Rather electrifying when you think about it.

A spirited discussion regarding the evils of factory farming cannot convey the sense of connection and harmony this path of non-violence gives me. I find oneness in nature when I see a blue jay or foraging deer and whisper softly, "It's okay, it is your spectacular beauty, not your flesh that sustains me."

The compassion born from veganism opened my eyes to the sanctity of our furry four-footed, scaled, and feathered kin to whom we are all intimately connected. Participation in the abuse and animal husbandry slavery blinds us from the brilliance, beauty, feelings and intelligence of those who man arrogantly enslaves. By electing not to participate in industrial animal abuse, we are instantly free to be awestruck by the depths of a cow's eyes, rapt by the fluid artistry of fish in their watery world, to be blissfully filled with unconditional love and magic for all life. It's within this that my plant-based diet became rooted.

In 2010, according to the Food and Agriculture Organization (FAO), whose mandate is to insure that people have regular access to enough high-quality food to lead active, healthy lives, nearly 10.2 billion animals were raised and killed for food in the U.S. But precious few humans make the conscious connection between this slaughter and various meat products that appear on their plates. The problem in the West isn't about eating burgers, it's eating too many of them. Half the world is dying of not enough quality food and the other half is killing itself with gluttonous super-size gusto. No wonder the rest of the world hates Americans. Alas, without rebooted nutritional literacy, take out the burgers and they will simply eat too much of something else like pizza, the new vegetable.

Factory farms are hellish. Screaming animals are stunned by hammer blows, electric shock, or concussion guns. Quite conscious of what is happening, most critters frantically struggle, anticipating being barbarically eviscerated while still alive. I'm no wimp. I've lived on the mean streets of Back Bay Boston where I saw people beaten unconscious, watched junkies OD and had my ass handed to me on a platter many times. But observing a slaughterhouse blew me away, overwhelmed by heartache and empathetic pain. After watching how animals suffer in factory farms, I knew I would never again harm an animal. Man's cruelty to animals laid the groundwork for my commitment to vegetarianism and veganism. Mahatma Gandhi said, *"I do feel that spiritual progress does demand at some stage, that we should cease to kill our fellow creatures for the satisfaction of our bodily needs."*

Underneath the fight for animal rights, my righteously angry fist shakes at the blood-stained killing floors, under my sorrow and pain resulting from the reality of cruelty and separation beneath all this. My refreshed spiritual journey inspired me to seek a food source not made of violence, greed or shed tears, but of love, awe, compassion and infinite respect for all creations of our mutual Great Spirit.

Every journey has challenges, and I've often pounded my balding head against the wall of confusion. I get discouraged and lose my 'oneness' as I journey along this path that so easily connects me to the life pulse of nature, and can so easily alienate me from my fellow man who sees my lifestyle as "radically strange." I become clumsy, inadequate, noticeably unenlightened as my heart, overflowing with compassion, becomes that clinched, angry fist. Here lies the enigma, "In a world gone mad, filled with anger, ego, greed and aggression, how do I walk this walk. How do I live this life in a state of peace and love?" Indeed, suffering is a part of life, though I chose not to intentionally watch it. Meditation helps.

Sadly, most have been wrongly brainwashed to accept animals have no soul because it makes it so much easier to butcher and eat them. An analogy means drawing a conclusion by finding many points of similarity. The animal is eating, you are eating. The animal is sleeping, you are sleeping. It is defending, you are defending. The animal is having sex, you are having sex. The animals have children, you have children. They have a living place, you have a living place. You dream, they dream. The animal recognizes fairness, we recognize fairness. Faunae express joy and happiness, we express joy and happiness. If the animal is cut, there is blood; if your body is cut, there is blood. Clearly there are similarities, so who are we to deny this one similarity-- the presence of a soul?

This indigenous Hoosier is an eternally grateful survivor of terminal viral heart disease, congestive heart failure, atrial fib, indolence, nutritional ignorance and obesity. My past liquor-drenched lifestyle and gluttonous All-American menu of dead food was booze, cigarettes, a big skunky fatty, and a balanced diet of Crispy Crèmes and Mt. Dew chased with unctuous buckets of icky KFC where the only thing missing is "U." Like everyone else, I grew up during the time in America when the quality and source of food was inconsequential and junk food supremacy was bourgeoning. My unexercised, flabby heart muscle giggled like Jell-0 in an earthquake. I was then, in the megalomaniac electro cardiologist's nonchalant tone I was brusquely informed, "Get prepared, you're going to die. Gather up the family. After the curtly delivered information re-enforced during daily rounds by my heartless, electro-cardiologist I was going to die, he would look at his watch, implying, "die…and the sooner the better." A molecule of hope would have been the best medicine, but he was too drunkenly self-centered and totally disconnected from compassion, kindness and love for his fellow man. Ego is good in small doses, but shouldn't control or mold you.

After a big ole' bowl of fresh gumption, I took charge, remained positive, grateful, laughed a lot, performed mind-body visualization, prayed to my god, and then told the ego-driven doctor not to return without a smile and a dose of hope. In the end, I walked out of the Cardiac Ward two weeks later completely healed; an honest-to-gosh miracle. The Cosmos wasn't finished with this clueless lost sheep and decided to catch my corpulent attention with an effective thwack upside the head with the Divine 2 X 4. In review, my disguised blessing came as no surprise: at seven pounds, seven ounces, I came screaming into the world during seventh hour of the seventh day, the son of a seventh son. What the seven's mean is yet to be determined. I'd say it brought me the luck for a rare second chance.

My necessary dalliance with the Grim Reaper illuminated why I'm here: mission revealed. Pudgy me, I promptly joined a gym, gave up dead fast food and cheese first, learned to like fresh, living produce, lost 100 heart-straining pounds, and then proceeded to turn the results of suffering into a career. I gradually evolved into a vegetarian, then a 90% vegan with rawist tendencies and proceeded to author three cookbooks crammed full of sagacious dietary advice, attitude, encouragement, love and simple recipes. Rebooted, I fell in to writing a syndicated weekly, award-garnering health column, travel around the U.S. as a corporate dietary motivator, teaching the spirituality, joy and bliss of vegetarian, vegan, and raw cooking. Since 2004, I've written content for and hosted *Eat Right Now* on WISH TV, Indianapolis. Providence?

Every cell of my being believes it's everyone's right to feel good, to achieve ones highest potential right now. Health is your birthright, your first freedom. Food choices can positively or negatively change one's life plus the surrounding flora and fauna. *"Eat Right Now"* offers up lucid, moral, non-violent, compassionate solutions, modern food science, hilarious anecdotes and inconceivable exposés regarding what's been perpetrated to your brand name foods, and the history of food as medicine for open minded CEOs, employees, responsible homemakers and parents. My lectures address that fresh, living, highly vibrational food was gifted to humans by the Great Creator for sustenance, maintenance, and to heighten spiritual connectivity and growth. In its place disconnected America's been trained to disrespect their Temple, the only home of the soul in this life, like a besotted rock star trashes a hotel room.

At work or play, are you brain-dead like you're awash in Jell-O? Do your eyes cross so much you want to nap after a heavy lunch? Are the competition and promotions passing you by? Too pooped and stressed to effectively socialize? Is that what harshens your mellow? Then it's time to revisit the quality and source of what you place into your often indiscriminant pie hole. After all, it's proven you become what you absorb from the food you place into it, garbage in-garbage out. Food becomes a physical part of your Temple: who and what you are. I don't recall eating a bowl of Sexy Beast this morning, however. All food fare, whether industrially processed or living and whole, leaves an imprint inside your internal wilderness. How you feel at this very moment is the result of your last meal.

Chef Wendell will visit your social organization, school, or business, shake things up, and enlighten employees and students by explaining how their innocent food choices affects their mental acuity, physical beauty, sexual performance, connection to a higher source, decision making, job safety, energy levels, and absenteeism, costing American business billions of dollars per annum. Many awakened CEO's already recognize the value of observing their employees daily choices because they know what they eat profoundly affects their health and safety performance at work, play, and at home. Your mood is in the food.

Today, after 16 years of catering for the NBA charters, I've witnessed firsthand, the anecdotal nutritional reality: teams with consistent winning records and championships are keenly mindful that food quality and physical / mental performances are deeply connected. Most significantly, I'll explain in layman's terms how the beloved American diet of dead, processed, genetically bastardized food profoundly disaffects mind, body, careers, spiritual connection and self-esteem. Safety-oriented, healthy, happy, congenial, non-aggressive employees lowers insurance premiums, creates less attrition and a healthy bottom line, an investment into their collective health, financial stability and the start of rebuilding a once great country.

I take my cosmic mission seriously, but it's seasoned liberally with levity, encouragement, hope, love, compassion and informative facts about the origins of food and the importance of eating honest, wholesome sustenance our loving Creator meant for us to consume.

"Let medicine be thy food and food be thy medicine".
Hippocrates, the Father of Medicine, 400 BC

2
Community: The Casserole of Life

After overcoming terminal heart disease, I gradually eased back into society and soon discovered my true friends. I was pleasantly pleased by those left standing: my loyal, loving family, members of my village, loyal business peers, and some colleagues. Most chef peers dumped me when they learned I gave up meat, cigarettes and boozing, and lost 100 belt-busting pounds. It's been accepted no one trusts a skinny, sober chef.

Call me an idealistic, people-pleasing Pollyanna, but I love my fellow earthlings and cherish spending social time with family and community, kibitzing, hugging, eating, cooking, learning about life, sharing, bragging, holding court, re-telling bad jokes, networking, and being genuinely involved in their needs, concerns, and contributions to our mutual village. We can all agree socializing in a pleasant environment of like minds makes humans happier and healthier. The madcap, imperfect human animal is transformed by mingling and associating with other humans. The socializing role of community is also important to the health, peace, and sanity of our teetering civilization.

"Sense of community" seems to be on everyone's lips these days. Do you recognize the valuable services within your community and treasure their contributions that support your family's physical well-being, mental health, piety, the quality of their lifestyle, and ultimately, peace of mind? My personal social and business community is one large, extended pack, and that's something quite extraordinary. Where would we be without our eco-friendly, family farm produce stands, early-rising dairy farmers, brilliant artisans, nocturnal delivery trucks, brimming with vibrant fresh produce, our dentists who nag at us to floss, the smiling jeweler, the local coffee house barista, the jovial spirits merchants who sell the red wine that keeps your cholesterol ratio in check and your tongue loose, the trusted family physician, and gym rats at your health club where we sweat and schmooze? Each affects mental, spiritual, physical growth and your groovy vibration.

Laughter is outstanding food for the soul. Hearty laughter gives lungs and hearts a workout, strengthens immune systems, and may help lower blood pressure. In this crazy, stressful, yet gorgeous green world, it's vitally relevant to nurture our sense of humor and personal integrity and then back away from engaging in anything negative that waters down our sense of community. It's eternally healthy to laugh at yourself and not take your bad self so seriously. Sorry, it's not always about you.

Lastly, who doesn't want to identify with the winning, excitement, entertainment, and pride offered by powerfully-built, role model thoroughbreds that play sports? The teamwork and pride of participating in special community sports programs or attending a grade school, high school, college, or professional game is powerful stress relief. Cheer, scream, shout, and let it all out! Its primal therapy to let steam off the kettle before it boils over or explodes.

I cherish my rich community of like-minded friends. Each is a part of me and together we succeed. Identify, acknowledge, and treasure yours; maximize your awareness and support their contributions. They're the essence of your family and village, the main ingredients in the tasty, nutritious casserole of life. After all, who we are and what we believe is the result of everything we've been exposed to, good and bad.

All thriving earthlings exist in a well-seasoned, structured, supportive community simmered to perfection for the good of the whole. Our families' glowing health is a teeny-weeny part of that success, a vital portion of any happy, connected village.

3
Cooling inflammation

From Alzheimer's' to vaginitis, inflammation causes 80-90% of all largely preventable disease. Continuous, uninhibited chronic inflammation is abnormal. Inflammation is a disease condition. It is the root of cancer, heart disease, obesity, diabetes, autoimmune diseases, painful arthritis and sadly much more.

Inflammation, your Temple's normal response to irritating internal damage, is your natural defense system to uninvited outside intruders. Authorities encourage cooling inflammation with real, fresh heavenly sun-blessed foods, not GMO, or the blazing conflagration of industrial strength laboratory 'foods'. You can only toss garbage into your Temple so long until it freaks out. If you drink booze, eat doughnuts, fast food, deli, fried foods, gravy, sugar, AP flour, lots of meat, and inhale environmental toxins and "Chem Trail" residue, but loathe glorious produce, you're innards are on fire. Inflammation naturally destroys toxic material in damaged tissues before it spreads. Autoimmune disease is a group of disorders in which your immune system attacks healthy cells in your Temple by mistake.

Obesity can cause internal inflammation which leads to cardiovascular and metabolic disease, according to the National Council on Strength & Fitness. Weight loss, though, is related to a reduction of inflammation, and the correct anti-inflammatory foods are the tasty answer. Invite spinach, kale, broccoli, and turnip greens to your diet. They brim with magnesium that relaxes heart muscles and improve heart function. Try about ½ cup a day, but if you're on Coumadin/ Warfarin talk with your phlebotomist. Green tea is a potent anti-inflammatory and anti-thrombotic shown to reduce heart disease and cancer risk. Bottoms' up!

Virgin olive oil's polyphenols protect the heart and blood vessels from inflammation. The monounsaturated fats in olive oil are converted into anti-inflammatory agents by the Temple and can lower occurrences of auto-immune asthma, psoriasis and RA.

Broccoli, cauliflower, and brussels sprouts contain anti-inflammatory nutrients which help your Temple rid itself of potentially carcinogenic compounds. Sweet potatoes are groovy sources of complex carbohydrates, golden beta-carotene, manganese, vitamin B6 and C and dietary fiber. Working in concert, these powerful antioxidants help heal inflammation in your Temple. And, wild-caught salmon contains soothing omega-3. Cacao, not cocoa, can lower blood pressure, reduce inflammation, reduce platelet formation, increase HDL and reduce oxidation of LDL cholesterol. Cacao vs. cocoa is an uber rich source of flavonoids, even more than tea and red wine. Dark chocolate contains more polyphenols and flavonoids than milk chocolate. Sorry, M & M's don't count.

Turmeric helps turn off certain genes that cause heart scarring and enlargement. Curcumin or turmeric helps to reduce the heart muscle and also prevents it from enlarging. Regular intake of anti-inflammatory turmeric may help reduce bad cholesterol and high blood pressure, increase blood circulation and prevent blood clotting thereby preventing a heart attack. Eat fresh, local, and clean.

4
Psssst! Want a free cookie?

Someone once said, about one-quarter of what you eat keeps you alive; three quarters of what you eat keeps your doctors alive.

Could you stop eating addictive fast foods, or do you need reality TV Food Rehab? Diets don't work. Education doesn't work as Big Food rejoices. As populaces eat slime oozing from the Western food cartels they've gotten fatter and sicker. Processed zombie foods, the greedy corporate predators that produce it, and indifferent government leaders are responsible. Around 85% of food you eat is processed, and the nutrient profiles of those products are determined by the Keebler Elves and detached manufacturers. Remember, if you don't recognize an ingredient, your exquisitely designed Temple won't either

Retired FDA Director, Dr. David Kessler discloses Big Food combines fat, sugar and salt to stimulate reward centers in the brain. They are opiates causing addiction like tobacco and heroin. You crave these foods and can't stop eating them. Sound familiar? You're not alone. How long will they repeatedly fail before begrudgingly doing something virtuous: after they've emptied America's pocket? A speaker at the symposium on Sugar, Fat, and the Public Health Crisis said the options available to policy makers and governments are severely restricted, but there's hope that working with industry in an ethical approach could lead to success dealing with a nation's disintegrating health.

Can we get all the addictive ingredients causing untold suffering out of processed foods and replace them with heavenly-sourced ones which will not harm, but benefit mankind? Eventually. But we can't change millions of decision makers' dark hearts overnight. All we can do is make better, more educated choices today. This is what this book is all about: providing you with dietary information leading to life-enhancing shopping, cooking, and lifestyle choices.

The only sane solution to transcending the preventable invasion of obesity and diabetes is for food manufacturers and un-lobbied policy makers to look into their dark hearts and empty souls, and agree to reformulate addictive processed foods with proper nourishment to advance our species. Yes, there have been slight improvements in the nutritional content of processed foods in recent years leading some folks to assume what we eat now is much better. However, that argument is a big fat pants-on-fire front row seat in a Hell specifically reserved for Big Food drug pushers!

Most folks don't have any idea how absolutely glorious their Temple is designed to feel each moment. Use natural substitutes for addictive sugar, grease and salt and put in wholesome ingredients like omega-3 fatty acids, food-based multi-vitamins, and vitamin D. The American food system has gone horribly wrong. But it can also go joyfully right. You can do it. Start from where you are, not where you would like to be and just say no to grocery store "drug" dealer tactics.

5
Is There Biblical Dietary Confusion

*Don't copy the behavior and customs of this world, but let God transform you into a new person by changing the way you think. Romans 12:2 ....***and eat.**

To a degree, we're all hypocrites. No one intentionally eats poorly, it's our current nature, and we do it with panache. Our imperfect humanness continuously gets in the way of spiritual obedience. The hardest part of living on earth is being in the world, but not of it, especially regarding your Holy Temple.

Manna from heaven was a cornucopia of delicious whole foods that sustained the people of the Jordan River Valley who generally ate uncomplicated, wholesome and, often raw meals. For generations, our culture also accepted God's scriptures as food for the soul. People of faith have obeyed scriptures, sort of, fearing they'll blaze for perpetuity. After studying various scriptures regarding our manufacturer's commands on food, I'm convinced proper instructions are there, but we conveniently diminish the message to accommodate our worldly pleasure-seeking nature. Look how we eat: creatures of convenience ingesting anything and everything a lilting mascot suggests, rather than obeying universal dietary law. It's easy to recognize the confusion.

It comes down to *Leviticus 11:46-47*: "This is the law regarding the animal, and the bird, and every living thing that moves in the waters, and everything that swarms on the earth, to make a distinction between the unclean and the clean, and between the edible creature and the creature not to be consumed". Judaism's kosher laws of the Kashrut are observed if food is made unclean, still with blood, or altered from creation's original state.

The filthy Western diet defines unclean food. Ruminant, vegetarian cows were created to eat grass. Today they're fed corn as well as other dead cows. Cannibalism? The advent of "mad cow" disease (also known as bovine spongiform encephalopathy or BSE) raised international concern about the safety of feeding dead cattle to vegetarian cattle. Since the discovery of mad cow disease in the United States, the federal government has taken some action to restrict the parts of cattle that can be fed back to cattle. Pretty sick wouldn't you say?

Our colorful grocery produce is 80% genetically modified organisms (GMO), diminished in sacred cosmic, healing nourishment and potential vibrating energy. Processed junk foods contain dead preservatives, pink slime, excess sodium, MSG, hormones, antibiotics, insecticides, food colorings, and succulent carbon monoxide. Big Food takes dark pride and giddy happiness in destroying Creation's gifts for profit, posing the scriptural query, "What does it avail a man to gain a fortune and lose his soul?"

Creation eagerly makes food for the birds, but does not feed them individually via a robotic drive-thru. Intuitively birds and all animals know where, how, when and what to eat. Americans prefer to be told. When I eat mindfully, I reconnect with nature's bounteous apothecary as well as my whispering soul. Suddenly, my Holy Temple and Creator vibrates in dizzy joy and thrives physically and spiritually. My straightforward philosophy: if my food had a face with eyes I can deeply look into, had a mother, or if man made it, I don't eat it. I seek a higher taste for my short time on earth.

I'm many miles from the mystery that awaits the end of my path. What matters is the journey. The peace and joy in the unfolding of self-found, as I let go of violence one step at a time. It's the understanding of the magic in the mundane that I gain as I make choices supporting the life force in all living beings. What matters is that this lifestyle we call vegetarian or veganism comes from, goes to, and believes in the soft unfolding of love, something the world needs much, much more of.

6
In Winter Dwell Within

In spring, summer and fall, mingling friends and neighbors engage in affable tete-a-tete. With its arrival, grey winter evokes a sacred privacy which no other season presents. Only during the chilly austerity of winter can one take pleasure in lengthy, hushed stretches to savor what's truly significant to the soul and our shared planet. In winter there's so little to do, you can permit yourself the luxury of fertile contemplation while percolating earthly lessons. As the garden peacefully slumbers, enumerable activities occur deep within the musky, sustaining soil. Just like humans, gardens use this time to process and stow away knowledge from previous seasonal experiences, time for rebuilding, reinforcing root systems, and for restoring cosmic vitality.

Most Americans still believe we have no alternative to the food contrived by agribusinesses raptors that care as little about our ecosystem and family's health as they do about the health of the barn animals so tightly packed in pens and cages on factory farms that the floor is scarcely visible, and covered in waste. If we are to survive, we must adapt and affect change. Every living thing was designed to cope with environmental factors like clean air, water, soil, light and temperature.

For emerging seekers yet to blossom, daily life goes on in complete disconnect from the adverse impacts their daily choices and activities have on the third star from the sun as well as the Holy Temple, our original home. Our collective minds harbor blind spots blocking our ability to see the fallout of contentedly suckling from the teats of Big Food and our dietary support of agribusiness eco-terrorists, a crisis of culture that has a gargantuan impact on all of the planet's flora and fauna, beauty beyond human portrayal. Happily, many developing greenies are growing more conscious how their behavior impacts how people live to the far corners of the earth.

At the commencement of the 21st century, society lost touch with what may be the singular sensibility fundamental to our survival as a species: a green, reverent, sustainable culture. Might winter be the time to consider how modern life has diminished our innate heavenly skills and wisdom? As the temperature drops, the days get shorter, animals, bugs, and plants have gone to sleep, the sun appears so low in the sky, appearing as though it will never return. In peace-filled darkness, we become more conscious of the wondrous unknowns of life, loss, death, rebirth, and the natural, soothing rhythms of life on earth.

Stoke a warming fire, sit next to the summer plant you befriended and brought inside for the long winter. Then reflect on how our species threatens to consume and befoul the natural world at a rate far exceeding our planet's carrying capacity. Scrutinize your life habits as you continue the voyage of greening life and home. Before the industrial revolution, our lives were intimately tied to the seasons and society developed unique traditions to express these transitional times. Each season had its own customs represented in symbols created for the celebrations; spring was about the rebirth of life on earth, summer about cultivation and fruitfulness, autumn about harvest and spiritual attunement, and winter was about the return of light in the midst of darkness. Dig into the reserves you accumulated during the year, a perfect occasion to bask in the glow of your imagination. Grab grandmother's afghan and curl up with your kindle, drift off to your favorite tunes, or journal your reflections perchance to discover your soul overflowing with clarity, like stars painted onto the infinite, cobalt heavens.

The initial tone of those cuddled up with the romantic "*Animal, Vegetable, Miracle*" Locavore mantra is "...how, in the dead of winter, can I obtain and prepare enough variety of wholesome local foods to receive my daily 40 or so nutrients required to sustain a healthy mind and body?" Patronize your local farmer's market and eat with the seasons. Produce shipped 2000 miles to your crisper drawer is a pretense. Premature harvest, mono-crop farming, and time diminish the life-force of the generous universal apothecary. This transcendence involves prioritization and creativity, plus a gentle nudge applied to your stubborn food perceptions.

Roasted sweet potato, pumpkin puree, or slivered earthy shiitake flatter steamy, wintery soups, stews or stir-fry's. Prepare a January salad of Hoosier greens with diced butternut squash, walnuts, Hoosier wheat berries, flax seed and carrots for additional nutrition and texture. Raw butternut squash or turnip "sticks" make lovely additions to a crudités of veggies.

Try a brussel sprouts salad. With a mandolin slicer or food processor, finely shred the sprouts, toss in toasted hazelnuts, lemon juice, virgin olive oil, aged cheese and then top with fresh thyme. Score a bushel of juicy local apples. Add unpeeled cubes to your Steele-cut oats along with virgin, raw coconut oil, ground flax or chia seed, walnuts, almonds, or pecans. Consider cooking oatmeal in a liquid medium of sweet, delicious apple cider. Or, at bedtime you can eat slices of apple spread with peanut butter to curb your uncontrollable sugar or milk chocolate Jones.

7
The Healing Duet

For years I dragged my feet, literally, regarding overdue knee surgery. Drained from limping and being restricted, I went for it and was pleasantly surprised how the experience has improved since I last endured a lost week in a purple haze of hospital food and constipating, narcotic painkillers.

My surgery emphasized the need for mutual participation to yield rapid, successful healing; you can't live life from the sidelines hoping someone else will do the work. To unleash the Holy Temple's majestic healing system you must develop a passionate relationship with fresh, real local food as medicine, as God, Thomas Edison and Hippocrates decreed.

Today, man conceitedly dissects food, removes the most vital parts, then, in false hubris, feebly recreates God's work in a petri dish when in fact it's the heavenly harmonious concerto of fresh pure nutrients that create the quantum healing power the loving universe unselfishly shares. Civilization's largest human tragedy is the priority of chemical therapy over fresh, living nutrition, the substitution of artificial therapy over natural, of poisons over food. Food, not considered medicinal by most, has become rooted social entertainment, pleasure, comfort, tradition, convenience, and a means to profit. We've failed to place food in context with disease, which is especially significant when the Temple isn't getting the right tools – the right nutrients which replace injured or damaged cells. Like rebuilding a rickety, aging home, quality materials are central to the outcome. Being nourished by food is the process by which your Holy Temple assimilates and digests food then uses it for growth, healing, and tissue replacement. The best kept secret in mainstream medicine is that under the right conditions, your body can heal itself.

"Are all these vitamins I'm taking, fresh local produce, and daily exercising worth my time and investment?" First of all, you can't out exercise a bad diet. Of course, you need a strong belief system since no one's handed progress reports on the investments into your health equity fund. Since birth,

Americans have been encouraged to depend on pharmaceutical drugs when they got sick. I wouldn't be alive today if not for Pharma drugs, though according to our Creator, fresh wholesome, sun-blessed plant nutrition should be man's #1 preventive medicine for all life. But that boat already set sail. Makes too much sense since corporate drug pushers cannot profit from what you grow in the family garden. Sigh.

If you've lost your appetite, a food-based multivitamin supplement with trace minerals is a must. Focus on zinc and iron for wound- healing and a post-surgery energy boost. Iron-rich foods include all types of clean meat and poultry, beans, apricots, eggs, whole grain breads, and iron-fortified cereals. Zinc comes from meat, seafood, and dark-meat poultry, dairy and fibrous beans. Other foods promoting wound healing before and after your surgery include locally sourced egg whites, walnuts, almonds, whole grains, and fish.

With my health priorities freshly rehabilitated, I kicked the Grim Reaper's scrawny, grey-green butt. Today I'm OC about daily exercise and eating real, unprocessed raw foods my cellular body intelligence can utilize.

When I fall down, I want to be able to get up. When I'm sick I want my body to heal. When I get hungry, I insist on and expect fresh local foods that heal; not what Poppin' Fresh suggests. Plus, I want to release my innate skills. Fresh, unprocessed plant foods provide your Temple with the ethereal sustenance that your 100 trillion cells recognize. This gives you the best chance to restore, rebuild organs and muscles, and soothe post-surgical tracks from the surgeon's scalpel.

Embrace your short, sweet, beautiful life with open arms. Stay positive. Take steps towards creating blissful health and create the legacy you wish to leave. Within you exists a miraculous universe of healing system with its own inner wisdom and deep intelligence that orchestrates all body systems in their attempt to fight off illness, heal wounds and ultimately return you to your original wholeness. For lasting healing to occur, it's necessary to heal not only the current disease but also the root cause of the disease, which frequently originates from the mind and gut.

Try to heal and purify your thoughts and mind, or the sickness and problems may reoccur. Remember, the Great Creator feeds the birds of the air, but doesn't conveniently drop it into their mouths.

8
Snack Attack

We spend over-busy days scurrying around in cars, running endless errands or becoming one with the computer. It is here that humans continually nibble on whatever's within reach. There are umpteen
reasons we snack: comfort, boredom, a quick energy fix, or just because of the desperate I-want-it-now-or-I'm-gonna-rip-someone's- face-off craving.

With beguiling vending machines every few feet, fast food and convenience stores loaded with bar-coded death at every stop light, eager to suck the life out of you, it's easy to be seduced by the fertile dark side of Western nutrition. If you intend to compete with the pink Duracell bunny, it's very important to eat foods that supply long-lasting, efficient fuel. A new study carried out by researchers from the University of Michigan's Medical School concluded that vended, prepackaged foods and sugary, faux colored beverages are linked to diabetes, obesity, cancer, ADHD, ADD, and coronary artery disease.

We're squandering a sacred opportunity to endow our family health and fulfill the divines' directive of personal stewardship. One way or another, everything we place into our Holy Temple leaves a footprint. As sure as I'm never going to have hair on my head again, you'll not find whole, restorative, socially redeeming fresh foods at a convenience store. I've seen freckled bananas, wrinkled oranges and pulpy apples at the checkout of a few, but their existence depends on the nutritionally illiterate demands of the local culture. Remember when they just sold gas?

May I turn you on to my fast food connection? Whenever the munchies attack, I head for the local grocery, waltz past the prepared hot food, then make a bee-line to the produce section where I grab containers of cut-up fresh fruit or vegetables. You may want to cut your own the night before to avoid the MSG used to preserve some pre-chopped versions. Then, I truck over to the deli for a container of humus, tabbouleh, sushi, guacamole, marinated olives, salsa, and some whole grain chips or wheat-free rye crackers. One day I might snag a small bag of dried fruits, bulk granola, pistachios or walnuts to keep within arm's length at work or in the car. Read labels since some granolas have infamous Trans fats. "All natural" fruit juice drinks and sodas, a meaningless term, can be soaked with sugar, a colossal contributor to a sick, fat nation. Really? That means cat poop is "Natural" too. I'm wondering when amoral authorities are going to connect the obvious dots between chronic disease and the foods they've encouraged the populace to worship. The truth is always the casualty of greed.

In short time you'll gain confidence as you note there's vastly more variety at the mainstream or whole foods grocery store, plus you're getting up off and working gelatinous gluteus maximus. Summon inner strength and waddle past the potato chips, gooey thingies, cookies, and fried bits. If you take time to read labels, you'll discover that major grocery stores carry healthful versions of your favorite treats. You'll acquire increased pep and mental clarity. Science has realized that eating junky, processed foods makes us "stoopid."

Besides what I've already mentioned, my favorite snacks are raw veggies spritzed with low-calorie salad dressing, Ezekiel cereal, Vegan Boca burgers instead of dead cow burgers, almonds, nut butters, guacamole, almond cheese, and rye thins, and banana bits dipped in dark chocolate then frozen on a sheet pan lined with wax paper. Zip-lock for a sweet treat recompense because you've been so good. God forbid you make air-popped popcorn from scratch. After all, it's so exhausting having to shake that darned pan while the kernels pop and ping against the lid. *Sigh*.

9
Water

Under a colander of stars, moonlit waters mirror heaven, revealing the intimacy between heaven and earth. Man is privileged to live on what planetary astrobiology considers one of the cosmos' rare, blue water planets. Nevertheless, man knows and cares more about the moon and Pop music than he does the sanctity of water, the life blood of planet Earth and its dwellers.

Clearly, man sees only what concerns him. Thoreau wrote instead of looking to the sky, look into the placid, reflecting salubrious waters for signs and promises of the morrow, referring to water as earth's eye; looking into which the beholder measures the depth of his own nature.

When the Great Spirit christened earth, the first morning sun rose, nestled within a soft yellow and raspberry sky and the atmosphere, land, water, plants and microbes were uncontaminated. If not for H_2O on the earth 4.5 billion years ago, all life would simply not exist. It seems anomalous calling our beautiful planet "earth", when it's clearly an ocean star as man and earth are made up of 85% water.

Perceiving water as clean, humans shower, wash clothing and cars, and over-soak manicured vanity lawns and gardens with fresh water. Yet most earthlings rehydrate their most holy possession, the human Temple, with rivers of frou-frou coffees, artificial fruit drinks, and fizzy colas. Assuredly, earthlings would neither shower in Diet Coke nor swim in a rippling brook of Mountain Dew. But then again, nothing surprises me anymore.

Of the thin veneer, life exists on just 0.003% of the total world water supply yet we take it for granted, desecrating the source of life with industrial twaddle. Consequently, very little of earth's water remains pristine. Earth's water is increasingly unusable and befouled by manmade contaminants. One of my two dead heroes I'd love to dine with, Thoreau, would be distraught, sobbing at the willy-nilly use of earth-poisoning herbicides to rid vanity lawns of highly nourishing dandelions, tiptoeing purslane, and constellations of flora and fauna. My other role model dinner companion is George Carlin, of course.

Slow progress in protecting water's integrity is not acceptable, as more than three million people die every year from avoidable water-related disease, and more bodies of water such as the Gulf of Mexico are dying. If man rises to meet this challenge, he must altruistically foster respectful approaches that are people-centered and earth-friendly.

Complex life is uncommon in our mysterious universe. Earth needs loving stewardship and prudent, conscious conservation for future generations to survive. Clean water should not be a luxury, but it could possibly become one. Water is constantly recycled and we all live downstream from some power plant, manufacturing facility or industrial agriculture complex. Healthy families, communities, environments, and economies rely on clean, safe water. To ensure our water resources for the future, we must protect them today. The tragedy in Fukushima illuminated society's agony of inconvenience when potable water is scarce or tainted. Remember we are merely guests here, caretakers. Dominion is subjective and frequently abused. In the near future, wars will be fought over water rights.

10
Harvesting Garden and Soul

With summer cresting, the solstice passed, warm earth begins to cool, days get shortened while shiny, plump crows caw over painted harvests, and compost-dusted gardeners and family farmers dance, sing and reap in joyful celebration. The third sphere from the sun freely yields what grows on its bountiful surface. The ultimate recompense of human bumblebees seeding, growing and reaping food, herbs, and flowers from Earth's gardens are to express, and create, then harvest beauty and nourishment with inspiration drawn from the altruistic well of nature's soul. The plant world lives not in isolation but in sacrosanct interdependences with our shared earthly milieu. Just as skin, bone, and brain form the whole of human carbon based organisms, edible plants are upstanding, indispensable human compatriots, equal members connected by our common oneness.

There's no form of food consumption more quixotic, satisfying, and soul-stirring than eating what's been recently harvested from a small garden plot or neighboring family farm. Not much fossil fuel is burned when plucking and reaping zucchini or sweet cherry tomatoes a few steps or blocks from the kitchen countertop. Green families feeding their clan from their sequestered vegetable plot squeeze pennies doing so. Diligent gardeners are acquiring gigantic freezers together with an eagerness to resuscitate the ancient mysteries of canning.

Growing, raising food and supporting the growing local farmer is an excellent way to obtain the freshest, most nutritious energy-packed produce, and often at reasonable prices. Wisdom decrees learning to store, temperature control, and preserve perishable plant foods. The American family throws away $500 of perfectly good food annually due to laziness and poor product management. Plant foods need a little help from their green friends.

Like garlands of pearls, flower buds blossom expressing joy by putting forth their delicate, aromatic petals. When a flower is respectfully picked for aesthetic delight, the Earth has a sense of well-being, for the Earth cheerfully shares its prosperity. For example, when the corn is reaped in the summer or when animals graze on the plant growth, fostering Earth has a sensation of well-being such as that felt by the cow when its calf suckles milk. A home filled with nature's abundance has extraordinary energy--a delicious vibration of love and respect. Food is sacred; our supper tables are an altar of gratitude to Divine Creation.

11
Food and Stress

We live in a fretful, complicated, yet stunningly beautiful world. When stress, a necessary evil, rears its beastly head, we're tempted to soothe our anxious nerves with a bowl of ice cream, a bag of fries, booze and drugs, or toss back two venti mocha "Crap-puccinos" in a row to hack it.

Zigzagging towards the fourth turn on the race track called life, there are numerous factors that place the kibosh on your health. Stress kills by chipping away at the foundation of mind-body health. Certain food and beverages actually add extra stress to our Temple, which in response creates cortisol that makes you crave sweet and salty food. Cortisol's a major cause of Poochy-Belly. A 2001 "Science" article determined that abdominal fat in particular expressed high amounts of the enzyme that converts precursors of cortisol into its active form.

Stress is caused by adjustment to a changing environment, ageism, bullies, lost independence and control over your life, fear of something dangerous, loss of strength and coordination, a lost sense of purpose productivity, declining cognition, or eulogizing friends or relatives over a casket. The knee-jerk response from doctors is to prescribe liver-detonating, addictive, hemorrhoid-producing, symptom- masking sedatives and anti-depressants rather than treat and heal the source. When you hear the ghastly side-affect disclaimers on TV, drugs clearly carry risks. Identifying what's causing your stress is the first coherent step in learning to deal with it better. Don't hesitate, meditate.

Comfort foods intensify physical stress. Chugging three cups of caffeinated coffee or Diet Coke raises adrenaline which worsens stress. Too much sugar causes tetchy moods, tiredness, and depression. Chocolate must be consumed in moderation. On the other chocolaty, gooey hand, it also increases secretion of endorphins; the happy, feel-good neurotransmitters. (One serving, dear friends, not a sugar orgy.) Living Foods educators remind us sugar and caffeine unbalance hormones, disrupt sleep patterns, and create fatigue. I also urge avoiding highly caffeinated drinks like Red Bull, (adding fire to fire) corn-fed cow butter, hard-to-digest cheese, red meats, alcohol, sugary chocolate drinks and non-organic coffee and tea. Eating cooked meats, wheat breads, gluten laden foods, and processed foods create odiferous bouts of audible intestinal discharges, bloating, brain fogginess, fatigue, and a clogged digestive system. When these symptoms arise, you're stressed! When you're not functioning on all six cylinders you can't effectively perform daily tasks which in turn escalates mental strain. When you're feeling groovy, you will vibrate at a higher frequency and stress levels plummet.

Sufficient intake of water is crucial. Seniors are often dehydrated but don't feel thirsty, while other times it's too challenging or painful to pour. Do your best to drink at least 1 ounce of filtered water, not canned beverages, milk, or coffee, for every 2.2 pounds of weight. At our age, protein is essential since it promotes hardy immune response and prevents muscle wasting. We should consume high quality protein such as local eggs, hemp powder, tempeh, lean grass-fed meats, poultry, and wild caught salmon. Fibrous complex carbs are a marvelous source of protein, too. They're in whole grain breads, Ezekiel bread, granola, Barilla Plus pasta, non-hydrogenated peanut or almond butter, quinoa and brown rice. Fats and oils should be limited, not eliminated; choose olive, raw virgin coconut, fish, chia or walnut oils, and fried foods.

Be compassionate; love yourself. Although the old gray mare ain't what she used to be, proper care and the right variety of vitamins will help pensioners enjoy a healthy, long life. Supplement with vitamins A, B-complex, Rose Hips Vitamin C, E, and Pantothenic acid, as these are considered stress vitamins.

Exorcise the tension from your Holy Temple. Inhale deeply through your nose and exhale through the throat with five slow, rhythmic breaths to relax your heart and block brain chatter. Then relax each muscle, roll your neck from side to side, stand or sit up straight. Step back from what's stressing you. A few seconds can offer calming clarity and perspective. Laugh because nothing relieves tension in your body or mind like a little humor. Sex is also good at reducing stress, although, you already knew this.

Even in later life, adopting a healthier diet, kicking stress and building activities into your schedule helps your body and mind bounce back from the effects of life's relentless left and right jabs. You deserve the best, because you are.

12
God's Private Garden: Farm-acy Time

"And God, (not Bioengineers) said, let the earth bring forth grass, the herb yielding seed, and the fruit tree yielding fruit after his kind, whose seed is in itself upon earth: and it was so. And the earth brought forth grass and herb yielding seed after his kind, and the tree yielding fruit, whose seed was in itself, after his kind: and God saw that it was good." (Genesis 1:11-12)

It's an old fashion, newfangled concept: the freshest seasonal local fruits and vegetables, raw honey, artisan cheese, wines, brews, breads, clean grass-fed meats, and bug-fed chickens straight from family farms to the family kitchen. I adore going to farmers markets, lively social centers where I always run into smiling friends and bask in the warm glow of community. These outdoor markets keep me grounded to the earthy roots of nutrition where fresh food fare is vastly more significant to health than the eventuality of a doctor.

Thirty years ago eating local was a radical notion, but times they are a "changin." Farmer's markets provide sanctuary from proliferating genetically modified grocery versions of the universes' creations. Anyone who sees this biotech time bomb with spiritual eyes will recognize that genetically modified plants and animals are not about improving quality or providing healthful alternatives to the world. They're playing God and polluting His creations. God's law doesn't sanction genetic alteration even though bioengineers proudly market altered organisms as something helpful to humans. The intelligence of the universe created every species to reproduce after its own kind. Thus, there's no reason for man to modify DNA and cross transplant genes from one entity into another. In false hubris, man creates species God never intended to exist. Such alteration of species violates the natural order. Do I hear an Amen!

Community Farmer's Markets solve the growing problem of food access regarding the plight of family farmers. Farmer's markets remind us fresh wholesome food grown without man-made chemicals contains maximum heavenly nutrition that sustains body mind and soul. As you know, to remain mentally and physically sturdy, our manufacturer expects us to eat balanced meals containing complex carbs, clean plant and animal protein, fruit and vegetables, nuts, seeds, healthy fats, and an occasional goodie as a reward for being a good steward of His creation. Nevertheless, we've been encouraged to depart greatly from the road of nutritional righteousness, mindlessly settling for what's set before us as long as it's effortless, and looks and tastes familiar.

Our grandparents didn't eat from the golden arches, they smoked non-filter Camels, drank hard liquor, decanted clouds of heavy cream in their hand-painted, porcelain cups filled with steaming Folgers mountain grown coffee and ate blobs of butter and cancerous bacon fat, dinner was either chunks-o-beef, pork, chicken or deep fried fish parts. However, they did not use poisonous chemicals and growth hormones and sure, some of the crap they ate was gross, but our grandparents knew the importance of fresh balanced meals and taking care of themselves in a much less neurotic, self-interested way.

What's right is often forgotten by what is convenient. In a haze of suitability, lazy Americans have resorted to buying Del Monte and Dole opaque plastic fruit salad cups shipped from China, Thailand, Mexico and the Philippines. Oh snap, the agony of inconvenience!

Thankfully, Americans are transcending this mind-set and increasing their intake of fresh local produce and backing off on meat and taters three times a day, and whole grains are replacing potatoes. Folks are returning to the simple preindustrial revolution lifestyle of their forefathers, foraging for fresh food from local farms. If Great-grandfather wouldn't have recognized it as food, then it's not fit for consumption. So, don't eat anything that comes in a box, tube, or bag. Breaking pre-industrial revolution tradition has proved catastrophic to the collective health of a great nation. The backbone of America, the family farm, has all but been destroyed by Big Food and "MonSatan." Let us all return to the sacred "Universal Farm-acy" and dance till the sweet music stops.

13
Fiber or You're full of it!

As a chef, everyone digs when I cook for them which often results in... "Gosh Darn, Wendell, we dug the tasty dinner last night, but what did you put in it? This morning, stuff came outa' me I ate when I was six."

America's backed-up my friends. Why? We don't eat the 30-40 grams pipe-cleansing fiber our Temple needs per day. We need fiber, lots of it, every day, but we're not getting it from the failed Standard American Diet. Like home plumbing, the 20-foot long organ needs an occasional Roto-Rooter. Alas, Columbia University says the average American consumes 12 to 15 grams. Personally, I never "Met-a-Mucille" I didn't like. Truly, avoid over-the-counter laxatives. Instead, try warm prune juice with two tablespoons of ground flax seed, the "Colon Pow" of the GI tract.

Did you know fiber intake is more significant than healthy fat intake? Fiber prevents the bloat of constipation, diabetes, obesity, digestive maladies, Crohn's, the heartbreak of terminal flatulence, and heart disease. The more fiber one "regularly" consumes, the lower the risks. A healthy, happy colon should flow freely. I once considered opening a health food restaurant called, "The Happy Colon", then Sandi pointed out the potential marketing glitches.

Fiber promotes bowel function, lowering your risk of digestive toxicity. Close your eyes and pin the nose; the average meat-and-potato, fiber-challenged person with poochy belly carries somewhere around 4 to 6 fermenting, decomposing, meals inside with no hope of immediate, pending escape. Visualize the status of food stewing, seething, rotting and creating methane at 98.6° for three days. Smellin' what I'm cookin'?

As a fibrous meal snakes through the intestine, it speeds thing up while scouring the intestinal walls of sticky waste matter, reducing the risk of colon-related ugliness. Look up John Wayne and Elvis' autopsies online. They crossed over with 35 pounds of indigestible fecal matter in their colons. It's TMI, but an acquaintance of mine shared she only greets the

"Poopatorium" once a month. Yikes! Bless her heart; her diet was a disaster. She refuses to eat anything but processed junk and reviles veggies, fruit, grains and beans. Grab the garden hose.

Digest this: fiber is essential for diabetic patients to control glucose. It causes glucose to be speed-bumped from the small intestines into your blood stream. Fiber holds nutrients in the intestinal tract, thus slowing absorption and reducing "up and down" blood sugar levels. For eight years my shtick has been every time I say "fiber" on my CBS TV show, a bell rings. Keep those bowls a-moving, folks.

Heart disease studies show a diet high in soluble fiber reduces cholesterol by 24%, reducing the impact of cholesterol on your arteries. Water-soluble fiber may prevent re-absorption of bile acids made from cholesterol. Fiber binds with them and escorts them out of the temple as the liver pulls more cholesterol from the blood. Water-soluble fiber lowers the total cholesterol without affecting HDL. This fiber also stabilizes blood sugar by slowing down the absorption of carbohydrates into the blood. Psyllium supplementation, in particular, improves blood sugar levels in diabetics. Oat bran, seems, is the most favorable.

Water-soluble fiber is found in oat bran, legumes, psyllium, nuts, beans, pectin, and various fruits and vegetables. It forms a bulky gel in the intestine that regulates the flow of waste materials. Insoluble fiber won't dissolve in water. Our bodies cannot digest the un-dissolvable parts of plant walls found in cereals, bran, and vegetables. The function of insoluble fiber is to collect water which increases stool bulk in the large intestine, promoting bowel movement. As a fiberlicious meal travels through the intestine, it scours the intestinal walls of waste matter, reducing the risk of colon-related problems. Overweight? A high-fiber meal fills you up for a greater amount of time.

Choosing whole foods can make a world of difference to your health. Forage for minimally processed foods from fibrous plant sources. Eat more fresh fruit and vegetables, peas, beans, wheat germ, nuts, seeds, ground flax seeds, quinoa, barley, whole-wheat products, and oat bran to get your fiber fix.

You're becoming more mindful of what you eat, how crucial informed food choices are to glowing health and reducing medical costs. Good job. This transcendence will provide you a "moving experience."

14
Sweet Potato: Vegetable Indispensable?

Aunts, uncles, cousins and nephews all salivated with Pavlovian panache and knew good things were in store when Grandma began shuffling around her warm kitchen, softly humming hymns and clanking pans as she lovingly prepared the annual family holiday dinner.

Other than the warm and fuzzy time we spend with our family, one of the remembrances is the annual gooey, sticky, artery-clogging, albeit yummy, sweet potato casserole. You know, the canned, candied sweet potatoes, submerged in a pond of melted butter, brown sugar, and finally feloniously assaulted by molten marshmallows made with corn syrup, sugar and confectioner's sugar, and gelatin?

Once reserved for the holidays, maybe we should reconsider the potent root vegetable as an important addition to your family's diet throughout the year. America's love affair with the every-day potato, a member of the nightshade family, has not crossed over to the often maligned, sweet potato, a member of the Morning Glory family, not to be confused with the yam, which comes from an entirely different species. And, despite its name, the sweet potato is not related to the potato. The tuber like root is rich in the health enhancing vitamins A, C, calcium, potassium, and fiber. The Nutrition Action Newsletter rated fifty-eight vegetables by adding up the percentages of recommended daily allowances for six nutrients (Vitamin A, C, iron, calcium, fiber, complex carbohydrates and protein. In it's report, the sweet potato scored an impressive 583. Its nearest competitor, a raw carrot, came in at 434, and the every-day baked potato, a scrawny 114. "High Energy" sweet potatoes also contain B6, manganese, and lutein, which have been connected with preventing macular degeneration. It would take 23 cups of broccoli to provide the same amount of antioxidant protection. It is clearly a super food from our loving and generous universe.

Sweet potatoes were a mainstay of nourishment for early homesteaders and for soldiers during the Revolutionary War. One colonial physician called them the "vegetable indispensable." This lusty orange root has saved lives in troubled times. The Japanese repeatedly relied on it after typhoons devastated rice crops. In the early 1960's, sweet potatoes kept millions from starvation in famine-plagued China.

Don't forget to scrub the earthy snark off your spud. Wash, brush and remove the field residue and "gifts" left by a passing critter. You can bake em, mash em', roast em', grill em', fry em' or boil em'. Change your food perception and enjoy its preparation. Turn the chore of roasting a sweet potato into a joyous, rewarding celebration of earth's sumptuous treasures. Do include them as a part of your family's seven to nine one-half cup portions of fruits and vegetables a day. But, you were already going to begin, weren't you? That's what I thought. Good for you!

15
Arthritis and Food

My dearest, achy-breaky, pain-pill-popping pals, you deserve relief. Millions of inflamed Americans limp and hobble under the erroneous belief arthritis is a natural part of aging. Gimme' a freakin' break! Again, you've been cold-heartedly bull-shitted. Millions agonize needlessly due to some uber bogus, not-so-erudite medical advice, and the slime of low-grade foods of the metastasizing Western diet slimes its way across the kitchen floor of tweaking, pleasure-seeking, and narcissistic American food junkies.

The word arthritis comes from the Greek *arthron* meaning "joint" and the Latin *it is,* meaning "inflammation." It can result from youthful sports injuries, aggressive autoimmune response, or by infuriating cartilage, the glistening white surface of bone joints. When this gliding surface is no longer intact, agonizing discomfort, swelling and stiffness result. Arthritis affects 46 million and is not in the natural progression of aging; rather, it's years of accumulated physical self-abuse, or a dietary deficiency resulting from feed-bagging the gory-awful S.A.D. of crappy, low-grade food. The reality is the inflammation pain of arthritis can be prevented, subdued, and aided by whole foods nutritional and food-based vitamin supplementation. Anything triggering an immune response also triggers disease-causing inflammation. Alien foods your immune system recognizes as not belonging in your Temple can ignite allergic reactions resulting in joint irritation.

The Nightshade plant family triggers arthritic pain, eggplant, tomatoes, peppers, tobacco, and white potatoes contain solanine which interferes with enzymes in the muscles causing agony in neighboring joints. Now, add red meats, egg yolks, dairy, wheat gluten, corn, corn syrup, sugar, flour, processed foods and alcoholic beverages to the list. Especially for individuals with Rheumatoid Arthritis (RA), the gluten in wheat, oats, barley, and rye are dietary scalawags. Doctors report a higher-than-average-number of folks with autoimmune disorders who are allergic to gluten. A new study also discovered folks with rheumatoid arthritis have a 50 percent increased risk of diabetes compared to people without arthritis. Get tested for a serious gluten allergy known as Celiac disease.

If you dig milk, butter, cheese, yogurt, or casein and whey in other food fare such as bread or milk chocolate, then you can potentially trigger the symptoms of your food allergy, in this case, arthritis. Allergy symptoms may show up hours or even days later, well after a food is absorbed into your delicate ecosystem. Bacteria, viruses, and parasites also trigger an immune response, so take a probiotic supplement or drink a bottle of Kombucha tea.

Since we're primates created for a mostly plant based-diet, many people have limited capacity to digest animal proteins efficiently as they age. So, when they eat excessive animal protein the Temple's ability to cleave all the amino acid bonds is limited. Hence, the proteins may not totally break down into amino acid building blocks, which leads to the creation of antibodies against themselves, a.k.a. Autoimmune disease. Over 100 types of arthritis are autoimmune related diseases wherein the body's immune system becomes led astray, attacking what it was designed to protect. For those with Autoimmune disease, everything you place into your Holy Temple is either making you healthier or sicker. There's simply too much research disproving the idea that the disease is caused by aging. So, get over yourself and ditch the, "If it dies, it fry's" mentality and god-awful foods from the guiltless, naive 50's. Sheesh…time to put on the Big Boy Pants.

Scientific reports reviewing 31 studies concluded fasting, followed by a vegetarian diet, is useful in the treatment of rheumatoid arthritis. Non-prescription anti-inflammatories include vitamin C, turmeric, ginger, cayenne and glucosamine.

Be mindful, it's never too late to self-manage and do use the conflagration of inflammation with informed dietary modifications and the no-nonsense use of nutritional supplements. Recognizing the relationship between diet and your symptoms can bring blissful relief. Go against society's dogma. Take the road less traveled by choosing the dinner fork in route to joyous relief, and you'll enrich your quality of life, shrink medical costs, and liberate your beautiful Holy Temple. You can do it. Life's too short to not to feel good with every breath.

16
Honey: The Other Vitamin Bee!

Of all the garden insects, bees are a most curious, organized and socialized set.

As you swirl an amber teaspoon of the nectar into your steaming Chamomile, sip on this: The average honeybee makes 1/12th a teaspoon in a very busy lifetime. Two million flowers need to be tapped, and 50,000 miles must be logged to produce a pound of honey. Bees visit fifty to one hundred flowers during one collection trip. Your steeping tea just became a celebration of Earth's generous bounty and mystery, in symbiosis.

Over 150 million years ago, bees were busy producing mankind's oldest sweetener. For at least 9,000 years, man has been collecting honey from honeybees. Self-indulgently, bees produce honey as food stores for the hive during the long months of winter when flowers aren't blooming and little or no nectar is available. Solitary bees appeared 25 million years ago and became social insects about 10 to 20 million years ago. Honey production is a willing proposition between the queen, drone, worker bees and the leading character, the horny, pollen-laden flowers. It's a very hard-working, well-organized society where insect and flower work to perpetuate the species.

The ancient Egyptians used it to treat a variety of ailments, such as cataracts, cuts and burns. The ancient Chinese covered small pox sufferers with honey to speed healing and prevent scaring. In Greek and Roman mythology, honey was known as "ambrosia," food of the gods. Romans used honey, instead of gold, to pay their taxes. Classic Greek text from Homer, Plato, Aristotle, Democritus and others waxed poetic regarding honey's virtues as good physical and fiscal medicine. Romans greeted their guests with honey saying, "Here is honey which the gods provide for your health. It is the elixir of life, partake."

Palatable honey was discovered in the tombs of ancient Egyptian pharaohs and on the walls of caves, prehistoric man painted humans reaping honey. Honey never goes bad since it's acidic, and therefore, not conductive for bacterial growth. The Bible mentions honey or honeycomb over 40 times. In the book of St. Luke 24:42, after Christ has been risen from the dead, the first food he eats is "broiled fish and honeycomb."

As a child, honey was a rare treat served on nutritionally bogus white bread, slathered with creamy butter. All I knew about honey was that when American Indians spread it on a white man's body, it was an efficient way to attract fire ants.

Honey is antimicrobial due to its very high sugar content, low pH and the presence of organic acids. It is used to treat cuts, scrapes and burns and to prevent scarring. Honey is a super source of energy due to its high carbohydrate content. Diabetics take note. Not only does honey contain the minerals calcium, copper, iron, magnesium, manganese, phosphorous, potassium sodium and zinc, but is chock full of niacin, B6, thiamin, riboflavin and pantothenic acid.

The sweetest of all, honey is chock full of antioxidants which defend us from free radical stress due to eating today's insane proliferation of "dead" assembly line foods. However, the less golden honey is processed and heated, the more antioxidants. Unfiltered, dark honey has the highest content. Honey may be included in a controlled, diabetic diet. But, Diabetics must comply with the medical instructions of their family physician 'on the take' from Big Pharma. Actually, I personally feel sugar should not be used in any context with diabetes I or 2. Why stress the pancreas any more than necessary? I've asked three allegedly prominent doctors why toxic, addictive sugar is not discouraged for a diabetic and I have yet to receive a gracious response; very cowardly, fear fueled and immoral. They sold their souls to Pharma.

It was the accepted practice in Babylon 4,000 years ago, for a month after the wedding the bride's father would supply his son-in-law with all the mead he could drink. Mead is a honey beer, and because their calendar was lunar based, this period was called the "honey month" or what we know today as the "honeymoon." Traditionally, after the lunar month concluded, the bride and groom would consume the traditional, "Honeymoon Salad," lettuce alone with no dressing. Tragically, I digress.

Be gratefully attentive to whatever glorious treat the universe will offer up today. The sound of the wind rustling through the trees, golden edged clouds bursting with silver white rays of sun, birds floating motionless then descending with ease to snatch up a tasty grasshopper....and busy, buzzing bees flourishing in a mysterious, wondrous world many of us take for granted. Bee Happy! Bee healthy! Bee nice to a bee and eat your honey.

17
Live Long and Prosper

There are countless folks freaking out over environmentally-caused diseases who seek ways to maximize their heavenly gift of health and longevity. A healthy immune system is more relevant than ever in our lifetime—especially for our children and elders whose immune systems aren't so strong. Might food be the answer? You bet your sweet patootie.

Americans are conflicted about one of life's most important necessities: eating. Corporate billions are spent fire-walling the truth from the public. They're conflicted about what to eat, how much, and the dubious contents and safety of foods oozing from the flawed Western food system. According to the American Dietetic Association, 85 percent of consumers say nutrition is important. Another 38 percent have made their diets more healthful, and 65 percent of people are anxious about obesity.

Lurking in the cavernous grocery aisles there's a plethora of diet *du jour* products eager to swan dive into your shopping basket, which, ideally, should be brimming with a colorful variety of fresh, unprocessed, nutrient-rich, living foods. Silly fad diets are cop-outs. The true solution is working together as a devoted family, avoiding processed junk foods, varying culinary customs to become happy, healthy, energetic, conscious eaters who incorporate variety, balance, and moderation into daily diets. How you feel at this very moment in time is profoundly affected by your previous meal. Your mood is in the quality of the food.

Most nutritionists assert that dieting per se doesn't work, since dieting requires constant obsessing and fretting over which foods to feed yourself and your family. That's no fun. The secret to healthy eating lies in turning food preparation into joyous family fun generously seasoned with daily, educated lifestyle choices and judicious shopping selections. What we learn about food we learn as children. Our loving children and grandchildren urgently deserve responsible, adult role models for a healthy future.

Sadly, Americans are addicted to convenience. In a time-strapped, super-sized world, many mindlessly over-eat all the wrong foods. We eat simply for the sake of entertainment, living to eat rather than eating to live. I underline that food is not just something to silence a socially awkward case of Borborygmi.

I grew up in classic Midwestern fashion where meat and potatoes reigned, and gravy is a beverage. However, abruptly in 1988, my self-destructive eating rituals instantly reformed after a detached cardiologist bluntly told me I was going to die. Trust me, the prospect of death is inspiring, so I took educated baby steps: so long to fried chicken, Little Debbie's, beer, whiskey shots, and cigarettes, and hello to the community fitness center.

Over time, I've become so much of a plant eater that I lean towards sunlight, but I didn't become that way overnight. It's a marathon, not a sprint. I've discovered if food isn't pleasing to the eye and nose, as well as the taste buds, no one will eat it. Therefore, I try to cover all the bases of eating intelligently when I lecture to social groups. My simple-to-prepare recipes appeal to a wide variety of skeptical, picky palates.

I emphasize the significance of eating fresh, local, organic farm produce that's pesticide and insecticide-free, eternally more nutritious and unprocessed whole grains in their natural, God-given state. May I tenderly encourage everyone to consider food as physical and spiritual nourishment and disease preventative; to discover the pleasure of slow, conscious chewing, savoring each bite and pondering its garden origin? Pause to give thanks and gratitude, and then appreciate the enticing aroma, textures and vibrating energy of a colorful, home-cooked meal. We must return to dining together as a family and taking family-bonding, after-supper walks where everyone can delight in the comforting, delicious flow of love.

Open your padlocked mind and drooling mouth and return to your original beautiful wholeness. Eat to live and offer never-ending gratefulness to Creation. Keep learning, and your Holy Temple will assuredly show it's gratitude by allowing you to live long and prosper. Plus, God will smile.

18
Sweet, Beautiful Corn
Summer Corn-ucopia

Dad loved Sunday family drives in the country even though his rambunctious three sons whined and fidgeted in the back seat of our '55 Pontiac. As we cruised, between cow-counting, we were mesmerized by unending fields of corn. Like windshield wipers in a downpour, in unison, our heads whipped back and forth as our young eyes, at 50 MPH, struggled to fix on each linear row.

Corn is native to the Americas, grown by Native Americans thousands of years before Columbus arrived to the New World. *Current World Archeology* reports new evidence the earliest domestication of corn was in Mexico 8,700 years ago. Domesticated maize reached Panama by 5,600 BC and northern South America by 4,000 BC. Over millennia, Native Americans transformed maize through special cultivation methods. Maize, developed from a wild grass (Teosinte), originally grew in southern Mexico 7,000 years ago. The ancestral kernels of Teosinte looked different from modern corn. The kernels were small, and not fused together.

Early settlers may have perished if the generous Indians hadn't turned them on to corn. Settlers learned to grow it by planting kernels in small holes fertilized with small fish. Wise Native Americans celebrated corn's health mojo. A one cup serving of sweet yellow corn contains 356 IU of vitamin A and 108 mcg of beta-carotene, along with lutein and zeaxanthin, powerful antioxidants that help combat free radical activity and prevent various macular degenerative diseases.

The average ear of non-GMO corn has 800 kernels, arranged in 16 rows with one piece of silk for each kernel. One bushel contains about 27,000 kernels. Each tassel on a corn plant releases as many as 5 million grains of pollen. In the 1930s, before machinery was available, a family farmer could harvest 100 bushels of corn by hand in a 9 hour day.

Corn's an ingredient in more than 3,000 grocery products. Pick up a can of cat or dog (carnivores) food and read the first ingredient: corn, used as cheap filler to increase corporate profits. Poor unfortunate critters. The real tragedy is that almost all grocery corn today contains GMO (genetically modified organisms), which has not been adequately analyzed by the USDA for future environmental and socio-health and economic impacts of grafting God's sacred design. We are the unwitting experiment. The problem of GMO crops birthed an angry tsunami following the U.S. Supreme Court's ill-fated decision in 1980 to allow corporations to patent life. God's word cautions against adulterating seed, or defiling produce. Deuteronomy 22:9-11 asserts fields should not be sown with diverse seeds. Man, in infantile false hubris, shouldn't bully the hand of our perfect Creator. Karma, baby, karma.

Seek community sources and farmer's markets close to home from a grower who has a faithful, moral obedience towards our magnanimous Creator's directives. Just say "no" to ungodly GMO's. About 80% of grocery produce is ungodly GMO. When a German court ordered Monsanto to make public a controversial rat study in 2005, the data upheld claims by prominent scientists who said animals fed GMO corn developed extensive negative health effects in the blood, kidneys and liver, and humans eating the corn might be at risk. Charming! And that's just one study out of dozens charging Monsanto with felonious chemical assault on the citizens of Earth Gosh, isn't that what Syria did to its citizens? Oh, I see, that's okay. *Sigh.*

The unbounded intelligence of the universe is the author of life and it's all His—it's His corn, His wine, His wool and His flax. Though we're allowed to use them, the ownership remains His and should be used for His service, not Big Ag. Karma is impending for GMO black-hearts for forsaking and not obeying creation's plan for us. Sermon over. Someone please offer up an Amen and pass the garlic-basil butter.

19
Farts: A Toot-oral

Don't say you didn't chuckle when in *Blazing Saddles*, Slim Pickens served baked beans around the evening campfire, inspiring a prodigious, albeit side-splitting cowpoke cacophony.

Admitting to it or not, humans expel ozone-depleting methane gas several dozen odiferous times daily. Not an appetizing contemplation, but, for gosh sakes it's a biological fact of life. If cheeky explosions didn't occur, my snickering grandkids assert we'd explode. Oh, the humanity! One friend suggests when terminal flatulence rears its odiferous head, one should seek a welder's job and turn a negative into a positive, but I digress.

Gas in our intestines comes from several sources: The air we swallow and the digestive gas from decomposing food that seeps into your intestines. Farts are produced by chemical reactions, aging food and unwelcome bacteria colonizing our sacred inner ecology. Understandably, gastrointestinal upkeep seems apropos.

Listen up, my loving bean brains, I'm not pulling your finger. You need to get over your uptight self, grow up, and eat some beans. Did you know the more you eat beans, the less you'll explode during morning mass? The healthy benefits of eating fibrous legumes far overshadow a temporary moment of social impropriety. Beans defend your digestive tract, as Roto-Rooter, extend your life. Plus, you might lose weight along the way. Some of the healthiest foods, touted as anodynes for cancer and heart disease, create the most methane. The small, miraculous orbs are high in protein, fiber, help lower cholesterol, guard against cancer, and are beneficial to diabetics. The infamous musical fruit is a tip-top source of B vitamins, including folic acid, which has been discovered to perk up brain power and possibly protect us from Alzheimer's. Pulses provide the minerals iron, potassium, selenium, magnesium and even some calcium. Beans are a good source of insoluble fiber, which promotes digestive health and relieves the slow-moving barge of constipation.

Loosen your sphincter; it's a fact of life. On average, you produce 500 - 1000 ml of ozone-depleting, room-evacuating gas every day. Eating foods with large amounts of indigestible carbohydrates like green beans, under-cooked legumes, and baked potato are hair-trigger detonators. Foods containing pernicious artificial sweeteners such as sorbitol, an alcohol sugar, also cause thunderous flatulence. Broccoli, Brussel sprouts, cabbage and cauliflower are also gas producers. Eating salmon, high in sulfites can produce a more piquant gas than normal. When looking at the broader picture, the action is imperative for living large.

Antibiotic genocide can cause people to break wind due to the lack of balance between the protective good and bad microbes which maintain stealthy gastrointestinal peace. Antibiotics (anti-life) indiscriminately cause good *and* bad bacteria genocide: like napalming an entire village of innocents to wipe out one bad person. The medical fraternity, terrified of Big Pharma, is resistant in recognizing their moral, Hippocratic responsibility to replace the good flora its annihilate since it's what balances GI chemistry and upholds immune function. After any antibiotic regimen eat lots of probiotic yogurt, Kefir, kombucha tea or a "refrigerated" probiotic supplement to re-colonize and maintain bacterial balance, hence, restoring peace and harmony to your rumbling valley. Based on the Hippocratic Oath, "First, do no harm," doctors who prescribe antibiotics should unquestioningly resupply them with a "Pro" biotic. If not, believe me when I tell you, your gas-producing GI and digestive system will be out of whack for at least one year. Fibrous fresh produce and fiber reduce the time food decomposes in your colon and the sooner the better. Imagine decaying food setting out at 98.6° for three days. Phew!

The Kyoto Protocol and a UN report once suggested a "fart tax" on cattle which could help tackle greenhouse gas emissions from erupting livestock. The report from the UN's Food and Agriculture Organization (FAO) calculated that the world's 1.5 billion cattle and buffalo and almost one billion pigs produce methane emissions equivalent to about two billion tons of CO_2 every year, or six per cent of all annual greenhouse gas emissions. Since new taxes are thrust upon us with regularity, let's hope it doesn't come down to this for humans who create

3%. Of course, I digress. Chill. Stop blaming the dog and invest in Beano and some tasty beans, the poor man's meat.

20
Gettin' Your Barbeque On?

For over 200 years the 4th of July has been a special day when Americans celebrate pride, patriotism and gluttony when folks fill their pie-hole with potato salad till the left side of their face goes numb. If that happens, you're suffering a stroke and need immediate medical attention.

With the understanding the Holy Temple wasn't created to handle so much food in one sitting, consider how destructive the super-tasty All-American foods used in these infantile TV gorging contests are to your body's mind-body-spirit well-being. Why anyone doesn't host a broccoli or spinach eating contest is beyond me.

Humans struggle to control what and how much they eat. Grocery store advertisers, not to mention reprobate food manufacturers, do everything conceivable and unconsecrated to make their dead foods look, taste, smell-alluring and melt-in-your-mouth scrumptious.   There's an inverse relationship between food esthetics and how healthy it is. Noticeably, the worse it is for your Temple, the more aggressively stores, restaurants and food companies try to deceitfully convince you it's mouthwateringly scrumptious. Ergo, the "con" in convince.

Americans use the Fourth of July and other summer holidays to do things to their sacred Holy Temple they'd normally regret. There   are   many   insalubrious   traditions   born   out   of Independence Day. Guzzling down too much liquor harms the Holy Temple, yet folks spend a day at the park beside the keg doing hand-stands with a beer bong, imbibing more than one would in a month! Let's see, there's alcohol poisoning, liver disease, brain damage, social embarrassment, drunken calls late at night, physical and mental impairment, stroke and heart disease, DUI, unintended pregnancy (oops!), car accidents, and STD's due to booze-impaired judgment. Yep, that covers it.

"Shey, hic, everyone, wanna watch me, belch, eat a habanero?" Many use summer gigs for fiery chili cook-offs. Gorging on spicy foods isn't necessarily bad for a person's health; the fact that it has become a Fourth of July false macho tradition to shelve moderation, makes it an entirely different story. There are perils for going overboard with spicy food. There's a connection between mouth-searing chili peppers and stomach cancer, heartburn, acid reflux, indigestion, diarrhea, upset stomach and multiple excruciating rendezvous' with the porcelain throne. The spicy foods people ingest at these eating marathons needs to be tempered. It's amazing how people subject themselves to agonizing heat to prove their manhood and challenge the limits of their taste buds. There is nothing wrong with spicy food in moderation, simmered with lucid adult supervision.

Distance yourself from the mountainous food buffet. Have a healthy snack before you arrive. Drink two glasses of water before having anything else to drink. Sit down to eat, chew each bite 20 to 30 times and do all the talking while everyone else is eating. If you don't want to eat something immediately, share what's left. Don't drink more than two alcoholic libations and when the time comes, know exactly what non-alcoholic beverage you'll switch to. To avoid the divine punishment, the hangover, drink a bottle of hydrating, restorative water as festivity progresses, especially if you're outdoors sweating like a contestant on "Wheel of Fortune." Unless you want to watch your liver swell from inflammation and explode like a balloon full of meat, don't mix Tylenol and alcohol. Share your plan for the day with your partner out loud, so he will hear you and then politely request him to support your goals.

I do not eat meat, but don't fault those who do, so my red, white and blue Independence Day menu ideas suggest a grilled local chicken and vegetable kebab, grilled vegetables tossed in olive oil and garlic, "fresh caught" Alaskan salmon, ground local chicken or turkey *breast* burgers, black bean burgers, chicken sausages, and a big ole' bowl of common sense and moderation. Make the recipe in this book for chilled salad of quinoa, diced veggies, dried fruit, nuts, green onions in a sweet, lemon dressing, or, gasp, actually make a real fruit salad.

Don't let the Fourth be an excuse for regrettable choices. Exert self-discipline and moderation; celebrate the holiday by honoring the nation's independence in a healthy and respectful way with friends, family and neighbors.

21
Turmeric: "Ancient" Breaking News

Got inflammation? Did you know the lowest Alzheimer's rates on Earth are in India where the ancient spice turmeric is used in everyday cooking?

Diminished and muddled in the biased stew of subtle bigotry slithering from the American low-grade food industry, turmeric's antioxidant and anti-inflammatory properties are powerful enough to disintegrate the amyloid plaques in the brain that contribute to Alzheimer's disease. Turmeric not only reduces the irritation, it also has anti-bacterial properties and can prevent infection. Pretty cool, eh?

For 2,500 years, Indian Ayurvedic healers used turmeric, a deep yellow-orange spice, not only in their delicious curries, but to treat indigestion, internal irritation, liver disease, arthritis, and urinary tract disorders. Turmeric was, and still is, used in Chinese medicine as a powerful anti-inflammatory. Hum? What did they know that we can't yet comprehend in the 21st century?

You eat the ancient psychedelic yellow, healing spice, also called curcumin, every day in mustard, curry and cheese. It flavors and colors milk drinks, dairy products, beverages, cereal, confectionaries, ice cream, sausages, pickles, relishes, sauces, and dry mixes. However, in these processed forms, it's a medicinal waste of time and money. After decades of concealed assault, i.e. Madison Avenue propaganda, a confused America strains to re-embrace the original, heavenly design of food as preventive medicine, the way God planned it. Instead, we're trained like lemmings to eat toxic machine cuisine for instant gratification rather than fuel, which fosters a healthy, intricate internal ecology.

Got the toxic liver blues? Dating to 250 BC an ointment containing turmeric was used to relieve the effects of food poisoning. The primary role of the liver is to process and remove toxins in the bloodstream, a filtering organ which produces 13,000 different chemicals and 2,000 various enzymes used in the Temple. An unhealthy diet causes your freaked-out liver to become inflamed, congested, toxic and sluggish.

Dig cocktailing? Curcumin speeds up the process of liver detox. Curcumin prevents alcohol and other toxins from being converted into compounds that may cause harm to the liver. It can reverse the adverse effects of excessive iron consumption on the liver. Before you do a liver detox with turmeric, consult a qualified and experienced integrative or naturopathic practitioner. My allopathic physician conceals his fear with insecure chuckles whenever I mention using turmeric.

Concerned about cancer? A leukemia conference in London established that eating foods spiced with turmeric, or in pill form, could reduce the risk of developing childhood leukemia. Curcumin's antioxidants protect colon cells from free radicals which injure cellular DNA. Mutated DNA colon cells form cancerous cells rapidly. Curcumin helps destroy mutated cancer cells so they can't spread.

Got zits? Turmeric kills bacteria and fights infection. It's considered a blood purifier and detoxification agent, which is an advantage in treating acne inflammation. It only takes a few days for turmeric to show results in acne treatment. Mix turmeric powder with unrefined, virgin coconut oil and apply the paste directly over acne inflammations. Leave the dried paste on your acne inflammation overnight. Do this for two or three days and find considerable improvement in the condition of your skin.

Got arthritis? Turmeric's antioxidant and anti-inflammatory effects explain why many people with joint disease find relief when they cook with it regularly.

Got Crohn's? This inflammation and ulceration, along the innermost layer of the digestive tract, can appear from the mouth to the opening at the lower end of the alimentary canal. Curcumin inhibits a cellular inflammatory agent called *NF kappa-B,* which has been linked to cancer, inflammatory and autoimmune diseases.

One caveat, however. If you take a blood thinner like Coumadin / Warfarin, be aware turmeric thins the blood. That's good, however, if you're not on Coumadin and are attempting to avoid blood clots, stroke or a heart attack. Turmeric, used properly, is good medicine. Its flavor is subtle and earthy. Sandi and I put it into tomato sauce, make yellow rice or whole grains, vegetable soups, smoothies, or add it to our green tea. Now you know what the wise ancients have known for many centuries.

22
Man Bites dog; dog bites back

Summer's gone to the dogs. There are dog days of summer, "spotty" or "stray" showers and the ubiquitous hot dog searing on the patio grill, releasing smoky-grey plumes of urban perfume. Ground and incased meats, mentioned in Homer's "Odyssey," hold a lofty position in the pantheon of American eating traditions.

Wiener-worshiping Americans eat 22 billion tube-steaks annually, but back up the ol' hot dog cart. Then, why does the American Institute for Cancer Research, the Cancer Coalition, and the Physicians Committee for Responsible Medicine warn folks to drop the frankfurter, so no one will get hurt? These well-regarded resources say eating just one trashes the Temple as much as cigarettes. Why, that's downright un-American.

Frankly speaking, it's not so much the meat, it's what processors put into it to extend the product's grocery shelf life, while ironically shortening ours. Nearly every grocery hot dog contains nitrites to combat botulism and preserve color. During the cooking process, nitrites combine with amines naturally present in meat to form carcinogenic N-nitroso compounds. These are well-known carcinogens associated with cancer of the oral cavity, urinary bladder, esophagus, lungs, stomach and brain. (The same animal parts used in hot dogs) Do not despair. There are local farmer's market vendors and a few mass-producers who proudly prepare chemical-free franks and sausages. You need to ask questions, read labels and politely request the store manager to carry wieners without chemicals. The wiener the world awaits.

It's true. Nitrites are found in spinach, celery and green lettuce. Nitrite containing vegetables also contain Vitamin C and D, which prevent N-nitroso compounds, so vegetables are quite safe and healthy and reduce your cancer risk.

For decades, hot dog ingredients have been the brunt of alarming urban legends. We've heard tales they contain snouts, lips, tail, brains, organs, ears, private parts, and other bits that didn't make the cut. Generally, meats used in hot dogs come from the muscle and organs of the barnyard critter. Other ingredients include water, curing agents, artificial coloring, delicious carbon monoxide, and spices. If liver and hearts are used in processed meats, the USDA requires the manufacturer to declare those ingredients on the package with the statement "with variety meats" or "with meat by-products." The manufacturer must specify which mystery meat, however. In the U.S., companies are required to list ingredients in order, from the main ingredient down to the least ingredient. It's the unholy manmade compounds added by corporate knuckle draggers that poison your tasty puppies. In Europe, the hot dog was originally assembled with high-quality cuts of various meats. Americans took a European tradition and gave it their perverted chemical twist. Meijer carries Applegate Organic dogs, and soy dogs can be found everywhere. Eat soy in moderation, however.

Humans are innate risk takers who take their franks seriously. It's your Temple, so choose wisely. The "You gotta die from something" excuse is lame. Wake up and seek the smoke from an alternative American fire. Tradition can be a double-edged sword.

23
Is Cheese Liquid Meat?

If, in no way, I ever see another pernicious blue box of instant macaroni again, I'll be a happy camper. It's pure shit for lazy parents. Read the ingredients? It should read whole milk, grated sharp cheddar cheese, chopped onion, salt and pepper, paprika, and another layer of cheese on top with a splash of more milk. Instead it reads like the ingredients to jet fuel. Where's the cheese? Make your own, for goodness sakes.

Cheese is a dairy food made from milk. A starter culture of bacteria is first added to convert some lactose—the primary milk sugar—to lactic acid. An enzyme is added next to coagulate casein—the major milk protein—into a soft solid, or curd, that consists of calcium caseinate and milk fat. Milk fat exists as globules of a triglyceride wrapped in a phospholipid-protein membrane (*Chemical and Engineering News.*) Did someone say triglyceride?

As 50's kids, on Sundays my brothers and I would eagerly latch onto a boxed "kit" of Chef Boyardee Pizza, turn on "*Victory at Sea*", then Dad and Bro's would grab Aunt Mary's afghan and snuggle together to watch. I'm certainly dating myself, but a home-delivered pizza during those blissfully innocent times was a rare treat. Pizza sure isn't what it used to be, however. A pizza today contains about 2 or more pounds of artery-detonating cheese on top and inside the crust combined with pancreas-stressing white flour, a cardiologist's dream. Got some chunk in your trunk? Don't get cheesed at me, but cheese is partly responsible for our epidemic of obesity in America.

Before the proliferation of pizza shops, Mom discovered the pizza kit at the grocery, and the only cheese was a smidge of powerfully flavored parmesan, not 2 pounds of shredded, gooey, mozzarella between layers and inside the crust. The gooey substance is loaded with saturated fats, catastrophic for our arteries and waist line. In Italy, only a hint of cheese is used. More is not better for our health equity.

According to the USDA, the average American now eats 30-40 pounds of mucus-causing, intestinal-blocking cheese annually. Cheese consumption has grown five times faster over the past decade. Burp! Never let the curds get in the whey of a good thing. Cheese is a concentrated source of many of milk's nutrients, including protein. Americans are pleading, "More cheese, please," according to a new study released by the California Milk Advisory Board of Modesto. Foods that cause constipation include cow's milk, yogurt, cheese, cooked carrots, and bananas. Anyone got any warm prune juice-my version of a depth charge.

The Nutrition Acton Newsletter informs us that Panera throws cheese on all five of its Hot Panini sandwiches and seven of its nine signature sandwiches. Gorgonzola, asiago, or feta ends up on six out of its nine salads. Applebee's was busted for applying cheese on five of its seven salads and all but two of its 12 sandwiches and burgers. It would appear they need to earn back our trust and take a course in ethics.

"Americans are eating far too much fatty cheese," said Margo Wootan, Nutrition Policy Director for CSPI. It's on sandwiches, salads, spinach, lean chicken, pizza, pizza crusts, and even on greasy fries. It's more damaging to our hearts than marbled beef or butter." You don't have to totally cut back on cheese. Did you know that man is the only species on earth that profits and depends on milk from another species? Pretty heavy, eh? Practice moderation, as you already know.

Seek low-fat, nutritionally jam-packed, creamy Daiya cheese. Yes, years ago, fake cheese tasted like doggie doo and wouldn't melt. However, every grocery now carries some tasty cheese alternatives that even fool my grandkids. We make grilled cheese, broccoli casserole, and baked macaroni with Daiya brand cheese and no one can tell the difference. Be lovingly sneaky. I assure it won't kill you to give cheese alternatives a try, but practice moderation. Unfermented soy, even edamame, is evil GMO nutrition that will not touch my lips. Visit the Weston Price Foundation web site for more shocking info on the evils of soy.

24
Cilantro and Heavy Metal

And, no, I don't mean Ozzie Osborne. Are you prejudiced against cilantro, the green herb humans either adore or hate? You might want to give it a break. After all, it was one of the first spices to arrive in America.

Introduce your loving family's culinary healing arsenal to the ancient herb which fervent detractors describe as "soapy." Humans either adore or abhor the tasty, ancient herb. You've eaten it for decades in your fresh Mexican salsa and Asian take-out cuisine. Historically, the herb is dominant in Mexican and Asian cuisine. A small percentage of earthlings called "super-tasters" experience a "soapy" taste that assaults one's senses like an asparagus farm outhouse. It's a gene expression thing. Cilantro, aka Chinese parsley, has an aroma described as a mix between parsley and citrus, and possesses a certain chemical that you can either taste or not. Coriander, the ground seed of the leafy cilantro plant seed, was the first herb to be used by mankind, perhaps, going back as far back as 5000 BC. It is mentioned in early Sanskrit writings dating from about 1500 BC. Successively, the warring Romans dispensed it all over Europe.

Hippocrates, the father of medicine, recognized its healing virtues as a gift of the universe. Medieval superstition believed it to keep demons at bay by chucking a handful onto a burning fire. Cilantro was used as an agent to combat Montezuma's revenge, for intestinal poisoning, to ease a toothache, as a breath freshener, and to muffle the heartbreak and embarrassment of terminal flatulence. It's chock-full of beta-carotene, riboflavin, thiamine, niacin, vitamin C, calcium, copper, iron, magnesium, manganese, phosphorous, and potassium. Green is good.

Heartening news has arrived via a Japanese study regarding cilantro's bonding-attraction for heavy metals, especially, mercury and lead. As part of the test, a group of Chinese test subjects had their blood drawn and analyzed daily. Suddenly, heavy metals began to appear in the subject's blood draws. Like actor Jeremy Pavin's discovery years ago that he was a human thermometer from eating mercury-infused raw tuna daily. The only change was the new chef replacing one who had walked out. You see, the new chef cooked with a generous amount of cilantro; the only variable. Case solved. Compounds in cilantro protect cells from the effects of heavy metal exposure, support liver function and a healthy, productive, evacuation as you take a seat upon your porcelain throne. If only it protected us from heavy-metal bands.

Embrace this exquisite gift of the universal apothecary as you add more Mother Nature to your favorite dishes like guacamole, salsa, bean dip, chili, nachos, tacos, or warm enchiladas, Asian stir fry, and garden salads. It makes wonderful pesto. Wash and chop it to garnish Asian dishes like stir-fry or a steamed fish, steamy soups, and sauces. Keep it refrigerated stem down, like flowers, in a coffee cup of water to maintain freshness. Add cilantro to sesame-ginger dressing when making a Chinese chicken salad over dark, leafy greens, garnished with zinc-filled toasted sesame seeds, mango or orange wedges, water chestnuts, pickled ginger, julienne carrots, cucumber half-moons, toasted peanuts, and tasty bits of free-range chicken that has been basted at the last second in spicy Hoisin sauce. Sprinkle chopped cilantro leaves, toasted sesame seeds and green onions on the finished chicken or vegetarian alternative. Stand back and get prepared to receive effusive compliments to the chef.

25
Hark Ye Vegetable Blasphemers

Are you a vegetable atheist who doesn't believe in sun-blessed produce, perfect human food created by our Maker, and has a stake in your family's diet? Breaking news! For those living under a rock, for the 10,000[th] time just this year, research says the connection between eating colorful plant food and the prevention of chronic disease is ginormous in magnitude.

Yet...under fear of torch-bearing angry villagers darkening my door, I pronounce Midwesterners vegetable agnostics. But they're not alone. The CDC reports only 26 percent of the nation's adults eat vegetables three or more times a day, and no, that doesn't include french fries. A downer considering the CDC reports: "When compared to people who eat only small, token amounts of plant foods, those who eat more generous amounts, as part of a healthy diet, tend to have reduced risk of stroke, type 2 Diabetes, some types of cancer, cardiovascular disease and hypertension. The benefits are crystal clear. People who consume the 7 to 9 "half-cup" servings of fresh fruits and vegetables a day have half the chance of contracting 14 different types of adult cancers than those who don't. Plus, you feel so blissfully good...whole again.

After kicking The Reaper's scrawny ass from my cardiac ward hospital room in 1989, I was cosmically moved to evolve into peace-filled vegetarian. People thought it was very strange and

I was vilified by chef peers. The more they laughed at me out of fear, the stronger I became. "What? You don't eat meat, you a commie or sumthin"? Today, a plant-based diet loaded with lots of raw food is widespread and considered the healthiest of all eating behaviors. It's trendy, hip, effective, proliferating in popularity, and here to stay. Obviously, the less you do to food, the more it can do for you. Plus, the rising price of red meat preserved in carbon monoxide and red dye is likely to push folks toward cheaper, safer, cleaner protein sources. But it's taken decades of gastronomic experience and research to get to the point where people at least accept vegetarianism as logical. Plant phytonutrients come from the colors in fruits and veggies that give food their vibrant reds, blues, maroon, yellows, greens. The darker in color, the better. Real, unaltered, intelligent produce contains scads of restorative nutrients and vital enzymes which assist digestion. Heat kills. Cooking living foods above 115-118 degrees begins to destroy its heavenly vitamins and digestive enzymes. For the most nutrition, raw food rocks supreme.

Yellow and green produce are sources of vitamin A, calcium, iron, magnesium, vitamin C & K and almost all the B-vitamins in large quantities. Eating more dark green, orange and yellow vegetables lowers the risk of heart attack, stroke, obesity and adult blindness. Instead of GMO corn and banana, help yourself to orange carrots, sweet potatoes, acorn squash, oranges, papaya, mango or grapefruit. Add arugula, chopped kale, watercress or finely-chopped broccoli to your clan's dinner salads. These powerful phytonutrients from the universal apothecary promote eye and bone health, support the immune system and improve brain function. Eating produce is also associated with weight loss, your mood, and a happy, clean colon. Green tea, ground flax or Chia seed, and fermented soy products also possess heavenly healing compounds. Grab tomatoes, red peppers, cherries, strawberries, raspberries, blueberries, cranberries, watermelon, and apples before chowing sugary, caloric grapes.

The generous universe blesses us with perfect gifts of health-restorative "living" plant foods. However, we embrace a fraction of what's available from the universal apothecary. Instead, the powers that run our country selected a limited list of produce they wanted us to buy, and look now at a sickly, depressed nation, quite bluntly, caused by malnutrition. These decisions were not based on what is best the greater good, just what's best for Fat Cat bankers and commodity broker's bottom lines. Sigh, greed trumps our health freedom.

As you shop, be adventurous. There are over 300 different varieties available today, so take time to look around at the glorious fruits and vegetables, each super groovy for good health and beautiful skin. If you don't know what something is, politely ask. There are two simple scenarios: eat with nutritional mindfulness to live long and healthy, or eat fake food for ephemeral pleasure and suffer costly, heartbreaking long term health consequences. You're so worthy of the best!

26
Potent Pumpkin Power

"O, it set my heart a-clickin' like the tickin' of a clock,
When the frost is on the pumpkin and the fodder's in the shock".
James Whitcomb Riley, 'When the Frost is on the Punkin'
{1833}

Call it melancholy, but when I think of pumpkins my heart travels to childhood memories of autumn as it marches towards winter; dark and rainy days, burning leaves, hot cider, *outdoor* football games, snuggling, hay rides, harvest moons, and of course, glowing jack-o'lanterns being set on porches by giggling children. Nothing compares to the scented aroma of a creamy spiced pumpkin pie hot from the oven and the perfume of a roasting, stuffed turkey, which genuinely implies a comfort linked to memories of life's autumnal celebrations. Back to the womb! But, do you perceive pumpkin as a food which could save your life? I doubt it. Alas, the only recognizable form of pumpkin seems to be the cholesterol-packed pumpkin pie and the front porch jack-o'lantern. Other than that, we give precious little thought to making pumpkin a regular part of our menu. The pumpkin's been given a bad rap. Pumpkin, the new kid on the nutritional block, is currently in the spotlight due to its high fiber, potassium and vitamin content which can improve the quality of your beautiful life and health.

According to research provided by Tufts University, pumpkin is a super anti-cancer food. One half cup of cooked pumpkin has over five times your quota for beta carotene (vitamin A) per day. Pumpkins may be used to protect against many cancers. Beta carotene also provides protection from heart disease and other degenerative aspects of aging. All right, there you are, frightened and looking a pumpkin square in the eyes mumbling to yourself, "Now, what do I do?"

Don't be fearful; try something new. The only daunting part of cooking pumpkin is the carving, cutting with a dull knife and an unstable hand. You can boil it, bake it, mash it, roast it, steam it, throw it at Ichabod Crane, or make soup, bread and cookies with it. Ever try pumpkin butter? Regardless of how you prepare it, the beta carotene, fiber and vitamins are "potent pumpkin power" and should add fresh ammo to your nutritional arsenal. If you cook any food too long at high heat, enzymes, vitamins, and it's ethereal healing mojo are demolished. Heat kills.

The conclusion you should be reaching is: orange foods are healthy, that is until we begin adding ingredients that make up most pumpkin recipes, cream, butter, evaporated milk, eggs, sugar, butter and especially shortening. You know why they call it shortening don't you; because it shortens your life. Pumpkin recipes abound. My favorite is to bake the meat of the pumpkin al dente, mash it coarsely like mashed potatoes, add a little maple syrup, some coconut milk, a pinch of salt, and a touch of cinnamon. A foodgasm.

References to the versatile pumpkin date back many centuries. According to the University of Illinois Extension, the name pumpkin originated from the Greek word for "large melon" which is "pepon." "Pepon" was nasalized by the French into "pompon." The English changed "Pompon" to Pumpion." Shakespeare referred to the "pumpion" in his *Merry Wives of Windsor*. The American colonists changed "pumpion" into "pumpkin."

Pumpkins were a standby of the early New England settlements and have been a revered part of Native American celebrations for centuries. On that note, a few pumpkin facts from our friends at the University of Illinois Extension:

- Pumpkin seeds, pipatas, can be roasted as nutritious zinc and protein loaded snack
- Pumpkins contain potassium, vitamin A, C, and B
- Pumpkins have more beta-carotene than any other produce
- Pumpkins are used as feed for animals
- Pumpkin flowers are edible
- Pumpkins originated in Central America
- The Connecticut field variety is the traditional American pumpkin
- Pumpkins are 90% water
- Pumpkins were once recommended for removing freckles and curing snake bites
- Native Americans used pumpkin seeds for food and medicine

Actually, oil-rich pumpkin seeds were valued more for their oil and medicinal properties than the pumpkin flesh. The Mayans used the crushed seeds to treat kidney infections and intestinal parasites, and the sap was used to treat burns. Early settlers hollowed out large pumpkin gourds, filled them with milk, honey and cinnamon and baked them in the ashes, split open, and smeared with animal fat and maple syrup. Might that be how pumpkin pie was invented? Speaking of pie, is the ratio of a pumpkin's circumference to its diameter called "Pumpkin pi?" The confusion comes from my math teacher who told me pi "square" and my mom told me pies "are" round. There are conflicting reports as to whether pumpkins were a part of the first Thanksgiving meal of the Pilgrims and the Indians or, as some documentation supports it could have been the second Thanksgiving celebration. Regardless, from that time onward, pumpkins have been and continue to be a wonderful tradition at the Thanksgiving Day table.

There are other uses for pumpkins only Peter the Pumpkin eater and Cinderella could appreciate. Peter must have been out of his gourd to keep his wife locked up inside one of them, and Cinderella, well, you recall, tooled away from the ball in a four-wheel SUV version. So, as you can see, the pumpkin is quite versatile.

Challenge yourself to add new and delicious, seasonal pumpkin recipes to your year-round repertoire. Pumpkin soup, pumpkin bread, pumpkin pancakes, and pumpkin bars are just some of the many available recipes. Light and healthy versions can be found everywhere in the fall. Pick up Vegetarian Times, Cooking Light, and Natural Health magazines for easy, family pleasing, healthier versions of your favorites.

27
Eat Two Apples and call me in the Morning

Eve had a devil of a time persuading Adam to eat forbidden fruit, however, since their ensuing expulsion, the apple has reigned supreme. In ancient Greece and Rome, apples were a symbol of love and beauty. Cleopatra was rumored to place one in Caesar's chariot lunch box before battle. The forbidden fruit was so prized; armies took cultivated apples with them into England and then proceeded to make applesauce out of the country. About 1629, both the seeds and trees were brought to America by John Endicott, an early governor of the Massachusetts Bay Colony.

Johnny Appleseed promoted apples as he carried seeds with him wherever he traveled, and planted them in thinly settled parts of the country; mostly for distilling strong-drink. As of 2014 America, the apple remains sovereign. Most Americans consider the white meat most delectable, not the skin. Apples contain a gargantuan 30,000 protective antioxidants. Paradoxically, the skin contains bushels of the heavenly, healing nutrition. Orchards of studies prove a daily diet of real apples, not GMO (Genetically Modified Organism), contain .78 grams of pectin per 100 grams of edible fruit, ranking them fourth in pectin content among 24 common fruits and vegetables tested. This only applies when one leaves on the skin, which settles the debate, "to peel or not to peel?": So, put on your big boy pants and drop the peeler, the skin stays on. The apple's soluble fiber reduces the amount of cholesterol produced in the liver, slows digestion, and the rise of blood sugar, making it ideal for diabetics. Adding two large apples to your daily diet is shown to decrease total cholesterol. Apple's insoluble bran-like fiber gloms onto LDL cholesterol giving it the bums rush.

Eating un-peeled, albeit washed apples reduces risk of colon, breast, prostate, and ovarian cancers, heart disease, type II diabetes, obesity, and tooth carries. A study on mice at Cornell University found that the quercetin in apples may protect brain cells from the kind of free radical damage leading to Alzheimer's disease.

Apples that rust have the most curative powers. Notice apples these days don't brown? It's because today's commercial apples have no semblance to the apples our loving universe created. That's because they're GMO, ergo, missing original heavenly components. What happened to Winesap, McIntosh, and Rome apples we relished in our youth? Royal gala, Fuji and the new generation of apples are man's egotistical manipulation of God's gifts to us. The National Cancer Institute reports the 30-40 K antioxidants in apples may reduce the risk of lung cancer by as much as 50%. A Cornell University study indicated apples inhibited colon cancer cells reproduction by 43%, and a Mayo Clinic study indicates the quercetin in an apple's skin prevents oxygen molecules from the damage that encourages growth of prostate cancer cells.

For your Temple to absorb the biggest bang-for-its-buck, choose locally grown varieties, which brown easily, such as puckery Granny Smiths. I gently encourage you not to substitute insipid, sugary apple juice for raw apples. Grocery store sugar-laden apple juice contains next to none of the beneficial pectin, potassium, antioxidants, quercetin, and colon-cleansing fiber. Instead, forage seasonal apples from your local orchard. However, ask the grower if they wash, sanitize, and filter the nectar to prevent E. coli or salmonella. Some orchards make use of the fallen apples because they are sugary ripe and easy to harvest, but pathogens lurk. One bad apple *can* spoil the whole bunch, girl.

Apologetically, the true "forbidden" ones, caramel apples, don't count. Add sliced apples briefly cooked in virgin coconut oil and cinnamon to your morning steel-cut oatmeal which you've cooked in apple cider, not water. Chuck in some walnuts, fibrous flax or chia seed, and fruit, and your colon will return the, a...umm...favor.

28
The Beauty of the Odiferous Onion Family
Take a Leek, Please!

"If an onion rings in the forest, does anyone cry?" As odd, whiff, honk...as it...drip, wipe...may seem to you, it's an onion a day, not foul breath keeping the doctor at bay. That's health news that should bring tears to your eyes. An apple is what you eat to clean your breath *before* you go to the doctor.

The National Cancer Institute has peeled away the layers to report that the 19 tear-jerking pounds of fresh onion the average American eats per year, scallions, leeks, sweet onions, contain antioxidants that help block cancer, lower cholesterol, and prevent a host of degenerative diseases. These soil-dwelling gems belong to the 500 alliums, which are thought to be members of the lily, amaryllis, and the Alliaceae family.

Apparently our ancestors weren't too far off believing the underground bulb is so much more than a lowly root vegetable. Paintings of onions appear on the inner walls of the pyramids of the Old and the New Kingdom. Mummies were discovered with antiseptic onions stuffed in their pelvic regions, chest, legs, and the soles of their feet and in the eye sockets. It was believed that the pungency and magical powers would prompt the dead to breathe again. No kidding. The Israelites mentioned their humble desert diet enforced by the Exodus, *"We remember the fish, which we did eat in Egypt freely, the cucumbers and the melons and the leeks, and the onions and the garlic."* During hard times, onions prevented thirst and were dried and preserved for future consumption.

The Egyptians tallied 8,000 aliments of which onions would relieve. Sixth century BC India wisely celebrated onion as a diuretic, food for digestion, the heart, the eyes, and the joints. The symbolic multi-layered circles of life made their way into ancient Greece where athletes consumed massive quantities because it would "lighten the balance of the blood." After Rome triumphed over Greece, the onion found a home in the Roman diet where it was rumored that gladiators were rubbed down with onion juice to "firm up the muscles." One can only assume that they stunk at what they did.

In Roman times, Pliny the Elder catalogued the Roman beliefs that onions cured vision, induced sleep, healed mouth sores, dog bites, toothaches, dysentery and lumbago. It had to be the antibacterial and antiviral properties of the healing onion.

Remember depression "Onion Sandwiches?" Thick slices of onion, jammed between two slices of Wonder Bread slathered with room- temperature butter, then sprinkled with salt and pepper. Unbeknownst to us, those stinking Sammie's Mom made for us were guarding our health with vitamins B6, B1, folic acid, fiber, potassium, and selenium, along with quercetin.

Onions, leeks and their other family members contain 25 magical, active compounds that inhibit the growth of cancerous cells, combat heart disease, inhibit strokes, lower blood pressure, LDL, protect against cataracts, and incite the Holy Temple's immune system. The heroes are not vitamins, but alliums, which incidentally, are antifungal and antibacterial. Two of these compounds stand out: Quercetin and organosulfides, both antioxidant phytochemicals that have been shown to prevent damage to our cell membranes.

Quercetin, a flavonoid, is an antioxidant compound that helps delay or slow the oxidative damage to cells and tissues of the body. Studies indicate quercetin helps to eliminate free radicals in the body, to inhibit low-density lipoprotein oxidation (an important reaction in the atherosclerosis and coronary heart disease), to protect and regenerate vitamin E (a powerful antioxidant) and to incapacitate the harmful effects of chelate metal ions.

Start peeling! If, however, you are planning on improving your health pounding down deep-fried, grease laden, Bloomin' Onions, it does not count. Sorry. Why, you indignantly ask? Each Bloomin' Onion from Outback Steakhouse contains a ridiculous 1,900 calories, 1,440 from fat. That's bloomin' crazy! "Stomach pump to table 3 please!"

Low-calorie onions are rich in two chemical groups that have perceived benefits to human health. These are the flavonoids and the alk(en)yl cysteine sulphoxides (ACSOs). Two flavonoid subgroups in onion, the anthocyanins, impart the red/purple color to some varieties and quercetin derivatives are responsible for the yellow and brown skins of other varieties.

Why is cutting onions such a sad job? It's not the pungent odor of the onion that makes us cry, but the gas the onion emits. When you cut into an onion, you break open thousands of plant cells. These cells contain chemicals called "amino acid sulfoxides," which drift up into the air, creating a sulfuric gas. You may recognize sulfur from the delightful smell of rotting eggs; a pungent stench that also burns your eyes and nasal passages. When the sulfuric gas from the onion drifts up into your eyes and co-mingles with your tears, a mild sulfuric acid is created! In response to the stinging acid, your eyes tearfully flush it out. It's very important not to rub your eyes with your hands when you're cutting onions and especially hot peppers. BTW: have you noticed onions don't make you cry anymore? Blame it on arrogant scientist playing God with our food with wretched genetic manipulation. Our Creator proclaims man cannot improve the cosmos creations. When man tries, he invariably screws things up and innocents suffer seemingly acceptable, collateral damage.

How can I keep my breath fresh?
- Chew on fresh parsley, but check a mirror before smiling
- Remember Clorets Gum and a green tongue?
- Chew on a citrus peel, anise or dill seed
- Slowly chew on a fresh apple. This also reduces cavities!
- Munch on roasted coffee beans
- Rinse your mouth with equal parts lemon juice and water
- Go suck on a cinnamon stick or clove

Let's not take the ancient medicinal root vegetable for granted. Eat with a conscious focus on your family's health. Then, perhaps, we need to loosen our sphincters up a bit and get over the misunderstood odor, and concentrate on the joyous, blissful, health enhancing, distinctive, pungent flavor of onions. If your friends are true, they'll accept you with open arms, not a clothespin on their nose. Tell them their idea stinks and, "I'd rather smell to high heavens than take a long, unexpected nap on the wrong side of the sod."

The 145,000 acres planted each year by the 1,000 onion farmers of America make sure that each American eats 19 pounds a year. That's nearly 380 pollutant-belching, semi-truck loads of onions in a day! Libya boasts the highest per capita consumption of onions at 66.8 pounds consumed per person each year. Pass the Clorets, please.

Onions are the favorite starter for many popular dishes and lightly sautéed, they add flavor. The professionals at The National Onion Association tell us when purchasing onions, look for dry outer skins free of spots or blemishes. The onion should be heavy for its size with no scent. One medium onion yields one cup. Be sure to cut the onions the same size for your uniformly sliced or chopped onions to brown evenly over a medium fire. High heat is the enemy and can make the onion taste bitter. Since onions are 90% water, please refrain from pureeing them in the food processor unless you are fond of onion smoothies. If you wish to freeze onions, lightly blanch or steam them first.

More members of God's magnificent celestial apothecary, scallions, Spanish, Vidalia, Bermuda, or leeks, are at most an indispensable, tasty food, and at best, magical medicine nurturing our Holy Temple.

29
MSG

"I begin to collapse toward the end of certain meals at restaurants," Jack said. "And frankly I thought I was dying."

According to CBN news, MSG adds flavor to your food, but researchers say it's also pilfering years away from your life. Of all the audacity! The MSG in the food triggered a bout of atrial fibrillation in Jack's heart.

In the late 50's, I recall Mom using Accent, the "miracle" flavor enhancer called "monosodium glutamate." It had become a household staple. We sprinkled it freely in every dish. I wonder if that had anything to do with my Dad's massive coronary in 1964?

Eating food seasoned with MSG stimulates the glutamate receptors on our tongue, intensifying the savory flavor of these foods. By the 1960s, Accent, pure MSG, had become a household word. Simultaneously, other hydrolyzed protein products such as autolyzed yeast, sodium caseinate, and hydrolyzed vegetable protein gained in popularity. Every hydrolyzed protein product, regardless of its assigned name, contains MSG. Read labels, please, my friends. Check out: www.trurthinlabeling.org.

Every food or food additive on the planet, in either raw or processed form, leaves its positive or negative imprint in the body long after it has exited your Holy Temple. Foods alter, transform, and determine how the body works. We frequently eat foods with dangerous embedded ingredients that sneak up and compromise our cultivated, nurtured Holy Temple, rendering you less than whole.

The first published report of a reaction to "monosodium glutamate" appeared in 1968 when Robert Ho Man Kwok, M.D., who had immigrated from China, reported although he never had the problem in China. About 20 minutes into a meal at certain Chinese restaurants, he suffered numbness, tingling, and tightness of the chest that lasted for 2 hours. The best American chefs, home cooks and restaurants, however, avoid

MSG and rely instead, as they should, on their culinary skills and the freshest and finest local ingredients that need no enhancement. It boils down to taste. It's long been known there are five basic tastes - sweet, sour, salty, astringent, and bitter. When we enjoy them all in balance, we become balanced, mentally, physically, and spiritually.

We're familiar with the Chinese Restaurant Syndrome. Many experts fault MSG for the reaction - the headaches, dizziness, rapid heartbeats and chest pains some people experience after dining at a Chinese restaurant. Some reports indicated that people with asthma became worse hours after they consumed MSG. www.chinesefood.about.com.

Since ancient times, sea vegetables were appreciated as one of nature's most valuable food sources by coastal peoples from around the earth. It's fuzzy whether the Chinese or Japanese first discovered that a broth made from Kombu seaweed enhanced the natural flavor of food. It wasn't until 1908 that Professor Ikeda of the University of Tokyo first isolated glutamate from dried Kombu kelp. Glutamate is glutamic acid that has been broken down by fermentation, cooking or other methods. MSG is concocted by mixing glutamate with salt and water.

Although glutamic acid had been isolated in 1866 by the German chemist Karl Ritthausen, it was not until 1908 that its flavor-boosting potential was noticed by Kikunae Ikeda of Tokyo, Japan. Prior to that time, our Chinese and Japanese friends used fresh seaweed as a preferred flavor enhancer without realizing that glutamic acid in kelp seaweed was the given flavor-enhancing compound placed here by the generosity of the Universe. Eating it in its God-given state, increasingly popular seaweed is a tasty way to intensify your nutritional intake, the flavor of your food and soups. Seaweed is, however, a hard sell to an in-lander. Do you eat sushi? Well, you're eating seaweed. Dark green dried Nori sheets, the Japanese name for various edible seaweed species of the red alga, are made from seaweed and are pretty nutritious. Give it a shot.

In Japan in the 1940s, glutamic acid was extracted from Kombu to make MSG. By 1956, when MSG was brought to the United

States in the years following World War II, it was manufactured through extraction from fermented sugar beet or sugar cane molasses in a process quite similar to the way soy sauce is made. Well, that's a departure that goes against nature! Sugar and molasses are not health-enhancing foods.

According to Dr. George Schwartz, author of "*In Bad Taste: The MSG Syndrome*," considerable money and effort were spent introducing MSG to the USA. In 1948, a symposium on MSG, presided over by the Armed Forces, was held in Chicago for members of the food industry. "Let's feed it to Americans and soldiers," someone suggested.

Many studies have found that MSG doesn't cause ill effects. Surprise, surprise! The biased "studies" were underwritten by Ajinomoto or other members of the glutamate industry, and most, if not all, were designed by Ajinomoto's International Glutamate Technical Committee.

Even before the Japanese discovered the flavor potential of processed free glutamic acid extracted from Kombu, kelp, or sea weed, the potential of freeing glutamic acid from protein using acid hydrolysis was being explored in Europe. At the time, however, the method was not widely used. The isolation, rather than keeping it in its natural state, altered it composition. I believe the whole is greater than the sum of the parts.

You're getting better at cooking balanced meals for your lovely family. Flavor enhancers shouldn't be needed when we can savor the tastes of foods in the state they were intended to be eaten. When you take your loving family to the Chinese restaurant, just ask them to hold the MSG and grease. Many Asian restaurants are already hip to the serious issue and have stopped using MSG entirely and deserve a tip of the hat.

30
Celiac Disease: Wheat's not so neat

Celiac Disease: 1 in 100 Americans has it, though most are blissfully unaware. Doctors are admittedly slow to diagnose the disease because Big Pharma has yet to concoct a drug for it, so it's not on their collective radar. They treat symptoms.

If your earthly existence depended on it, could you stop eating one particular food if it just about instantly reinstated your health entitlement? Wouldn't it blow your medulla oblongata if the guilty foodstuff, wheat gluten of all things, was the foundation of your illness?

"Do you not know that your body is a temple of the Holy Spirit, who is in you, whom you have received from God? You are not your own; you were bought at a price. Therefore honor God with your body," (1 Cor. 6:19-20).

Christians and most religions believe our bodies are temples of the Holy Spirit and should be nourished and treated ccordingly. Well, that one, like gluttony and coveting, got conveniently swept under the holy rug of religious hypocrisy.

Jesus repeatedly referred to bread, saying grains are the staff of life. Jesus even called himself the "Bread of Life," so how can eating grains be bad? Man's unbridled greed and arrogant disrespect for God, perhaps. Today's dead, toxic, genetically altered, herbicide infused twaddle is ditch-worthy. Why would you put something like this into your Holy Temple? You're trained like mice through aggressive advertising. Although it's probably easier to get people to change their religion than to change their diet.

Author and cardiologist William Davis, MD, says big agriculture stepped in decades ago to develop a higher-yielding crop. Today's "wheat," he says, isn't even wheat, thanks to intense crossbreeding efforts. "The wheat products sold today are nothing like the wheat products of our grandmother's age, very different from the wheat of the early 20th Century, and completely transformed from the wheat of the Bible," he says.

Alas, you're told eat to more whole grains, but most people still don't eat enough. In fact, it's estimated Americans only consume 1/3 of the whole grains into their diets that they should. 'Real' whole grains provide infinitely more heavenly nutrition than refined grains, are higher in fiber, vitamins, minerals and antioxidants. Simultaneously, researchers are waving big red flags saying Gluten intolerance, Celiac Disease is an epidemic because wheat, if you dare call it that, is hardly a health food. It makes you fat, causes gas and makes your intestinal tract your enemy

Personally I think God struck perfection creating the appropriate nourishment humans need to thrive and survive. Not sure the God I worship created U.S. to be the sickly bunch we've become. I mean, come on, how can man in greed and false hubris think he can second guess and improve on God's works? That's the mountain top of insane arrogance. When the unenlightened defend the wholesale bastardization of Creations gifts, under the salvation of feeding the world...really? Some third world countries are worse off after we dump off nutritionally bogus white rice and AP flour, "Look what we did."

Your magnificent, beautiful temple was programed to express perfect health from the day you were born. But it needs your help. Let's see some religious compliance and outrage at man's flipping off his loving, compassionate Creator. Check out: http://digestive.niddk.nih.gov/ddiseases/pubs/Celiac/

Wheat: Part 2

"I'm inexplicably depressed. My rumbling gastrointestinal tribulations, asthma, iron deficiency anemia, heart burn, low energy and early osteoporosis bring me down." Unable to connect the dots, Irma suffered for decades. The darling 65-year-old, bless her heart, couldn't understand why she was constantly bloated and cramping, flatulent, and couldn't summon the gumption to socialize. She already conceded her familial genes were responsible for her uncharacteristic early-life osteoarthritis. Not true.

After carpet bombing her innards with pharmaceutical drugs, her doctor tested for Celiac Disease (CD). Gluten intolerance appeared. One week into a wheat-free diet, she'd never felt better; she felt more human, joyful, and eager to socialize with her silver-haired homeys. It's startling how many seniors have undiagnosed CD because of wheat, one of the world's most important food crops. Her blessed relief lay right before her eyes.

Until the mid-1990's people didn't believe CD could develop in older people because it was considered a disease of childhood, "failing to thrive." Foods made from wheat and certain grains contain a protein called gluten. If you have CD, every time you eat gluten an immune reaction aggressively attacks your Vila, terminating healthy tissues of the small intestine where nutrients are absorbed. This leads to a cascade of health tribulations. Even teeny amounts of gluten trigger the response.

In her mind, she ate what she sincerely perceived as healthy cuisine: Raisin Bran with berries and walnuts for breakfast, whole wheat bread and lean turkey breast sandwich at lunch and, in between, some whole grain crackers and carrot sticks. At night, Irma ate brown rice, a breaded chicken breast with a dark green leafy salad with blue cheese dressing. Her absolutely favorite restaurant meal was a garden salad with croutons, pasta Bolognese dusted with Parma and more gooey garlic bread washed down with a mug-o-beer. Sounds benign however most of these wheat-based foods and beer contain various forms of gluten.

Irma is 1 in 10 Americans who needlessly suffers from the ancient malady, creating a high death rate when undiagnosed. Mayo Clinic research teams studied data from the 45 years of follow-up of Air Force subjects and showed those with undiagnosed Celiac Disease had a 400 percent higher risk of death than non-Celiacs. Two physicians I quizzed admit the medical fraternity has been slow-moving to diagnose the ubiquitous disease which shortens life expectancy--are you ready for this--by a whopping 4.5 times. It's curious contemporary doctors can't diagnose CD, since as far back as 250 AD, Aretaeus of Cappadocia included detailed descriptions of a disease he referred to his patients as kolliakos, meaning, "suffering in the bowels," which later translated to Celiacs.

A Naturopathic physician shares, "When CD symptoms *should* be the first condition that comes to mind, it's often misdiagnosed. Modern medicine does not consider CD first because, I believe, currently they don't have a drug for it yet." Celiacs get diagnosed as having irritable bowel syndrome, which in my opinion is a symptom, not a disease.

It takes two to four weeks of a strict gluten-free diet before you start to feel alive again, though some people get their mojo back within days. However, don't challenge your inner ecology by eating a large amount of wheat to see what happens. This is serious biz, so don't loaf around. You could end up sicker than before and this could cost you some serious bread. Gluten-free products abound at your community grocers. Not only is gluten found in grains like wheat, barley, rye, oats, malt and rye, it's also added to countless foods. For example, some ice creams and ketchups contain gluten as a thickening agent. The simple answer: read labels to avoid wheat products and foods prepared with wheat gluten often referred to as Wheat Meat. Mindfully place food and disease in the same context; it may save your life. For excellent information and list of foods with gluten: http://customchoicecereal.com/blog/.

Read recently published books and then turn to websites / support blogs run by Celiac organizations, noted Celiac research centers and trusted Integrative Nutritionists. Naturopaths suggest, "If you have any of the symptoms mentioned, simply eliminate all gluten-bearing foods for a month. If things clear up, continue on. Consult with an Integrative Physician and Nutritionist who specialize in Celiac disease before you embark on your quest for a return to wholeness. Sun- dappled vegetables, fruits, beans, seeds and meats are gluten-free foods." Sweet Irma factored her age and thought her diet was above reproach. Get checked for CD and free yourself. The simple act of transcending just one pleasurable food can be life transforming.

1. Identify your allergy/intolerance/sensitivity
Know which foods trigger a reaction and study the names they may hide under. Many ingredients go by multiple names, so if you think you may forget all the things you are looking for, bring a list to the store until you feel confident that you've got it (See the list below). You can purchase a listing of known gluten-free brands as a reference on an iPhone app or in book form (I use "Cecilia's Gluten-free Shopping Guide", by Matison and Matison).

2. Read, read, and read again
Even if you've purchased a product dozens of times, check the label each time. Companies frequently change their formulas in

order to save money, switch suppliers, or improve lagging sales.

3. If needed, contact the manufacturer

If you've gone to the store armed with knowledge of what you're avoiding, you've read the label, and you still can't figure out if a product is safe, call the manufacturer. Almost all websites list a customer service email or phone number, and companies are happy to talk to you about their ingredients and processes. Kraft bullies got suspicious of me when I called to ask what was in their faux American cheese slices. They rudely hung up on me when they heard I was a professional food writer.

Just because a product doesn't say it's gluten-free in big bold letters on the front, doesn't mean it isn't. Many products are naturally gluten-free and aren't necessarily going to call your attention to them. By the same token, I've spoken to companies who use a lot of legal mumbo-jumbo to avoid verifying that something is absolutely gluten-free even though it is because they are afraid of being sued if you happen to get sick. That happened today with an email response from a household product company. They actually said they will not say if any of their products are gluten-free because it is the customer's responsibility to check. That doesn't mean none of their products are GF. Just try to wade through the conversation or email and separate out the real story from the legal jargon. If in doubt, proceed to step 4.

4. When in doubt, leave it out!

If your reaction to the foods you are trying to avoid is fairly mild, you may be up for a "bite" for experimentation's sake when you are unsure, but for the majority of gluten-free folks or those with other allergies and sensitivities, it's simply not that easy.

5. Are Oats Safe on a GF diet?

It is likely that oats processed on the same equipment with wheat are contaminated, but oats in and of themselves have been found by the American Dietetic Association to be safe for Celiac. Do your homework (Bob's Red Mill and a few others sell gluten-free oats.)

Hidden Gluten Sources

Obviously on a gluten-free diet, the main grains to avoid are wheat, barley and rye, and anything derived from those three grains. Here are some ingredients that MAY have gluten. Some manufacturers will clarify the source of the ingredient if it is not specified on the label.

- Avena Sativa (Oat) kernel flour
- Barley extract
- Cyclodextrin
- Dextrin
- Dextrub Palmitate
- Emulsifier
- Fermented grain extract
- Flavoring
- Flour or cereal products, unless made with pure rice flour, corn flour, potato flour, or soy flour
- Hydrolyzed malt extract
- Hydrolyzed oat flour
- Hydrolyzed plant protein
- Hydrolyzed vegetable protein, unless its source is corn or soy
- Hydrolyzed wheat flour
- Hydrolyzed wheat gluten
- Hydrolyzed wheat protein
- Hydrolyzed wheat protein/PVP Crosspolymer
- Hydrolyzed wheat starch
- Malt or malt flavoring, unless its source is corn
- Maltodextrin (can be derived from wheat or corn)
- Modified starch or modified food starch, unless arrowroot, corn, potato, tapioca, waxy maize, or maize is used
- Phytosphingosine extract
- Samino peptide complex
- Secale Cereale (Rye) Seed Flour
- Sodium C8-16 Isoalkylsuccinyl
- Soy sauce or soy sauce solids, unless it's marked 'wheat-free'
- Stabilizers
- Starch

- Triticum Vulgare (wheat) germ extract
- Triticum Vulgare (wheat) germ Oil
- Triticum Vulgare (wheat) gluten
- Triticum Vulgare (wheat) starch
- Vitamin E (source can be wheat germ – clarify with manufacturer)
- Wheat amino acids
- Wheat germ glycerides
- Wheat Protein Sufonate
- Yeast extract

31
What's with Wheat and Soy?

Up against the wall, soy and wheat, you're charged for willfully masquerading as healthy while concealing the reality you're destructive to human health. We mustn't believe everything advertising pukes upon us.

Excluding toxic sugar, nearly 70 percent of all calories in the Western diet come from a combination of GMO wheat, dairy, soy, and corn. The problem: they're poisonous to our Temple and don't advance our health. Instead, these icons increase our weight and then short-chain long-term health.

When wheat, the sacred staff of life, was genetically altered to become semi-dwarf wheat in the last century, it was *assumed*, *without testing*, that the modifications wouldn't change how it affected the health of those who ate it. There's a large body of evidence indicating whole grains and whole wheat in particular, even organic, can contribute to major physical and mental health problems. Wheat is particularly problematic as a result of the wheat germ agglutinin (WGA) it contains.

Both ooze from processed junk foods and each is profoundly inflammatory, immunotoxic and neurotoxic. Over 90 percent of U.S. soy, including edamame, is genetically manipulated to make it grow faster. It's also altered so its genetic makeup includes Round-up herbicide. Yep. You're consuming lipsmakin', cancer-causing Round-up which pairs well, BTW, with a fruity, dry red wine. Just kidding.

Despite the alleged role of soybeans to a healthy diet, they're among the most common food allergens, reports the Asthma and Allergy Foundation of America. Soy contains at least 15 potential allergens that may trigger allergic symptoms and snarky side effects. Soy has a potential for creating blood clots. Hemaglutinin in soy may cause red blood cells to become increasingly sticky and clump together. These clumps are unable to process or transport oxygen as well across tissue membranes. Soy goitrogenan interrupts thyroid function and iodine metabolism resulting in long-term thyroid problems and hinder the creation of thyroid hormones.

Burly, manly men! According to 16 various research papers, soy kills testicular tissue. Soy permanently reduces testicular function and lowers hormone production that triggers your testicles to work. Any opinions to contrary have been paid for by the Agribusiness giants Monsanto and Archer Daniels Midland. Once public knowledge of their manipulation of public opinion becomes widely known, expect monster class action lawsuits against these love-starved street corner thugs and con artists. Karma's a bitch. Stick with fermented soy foods: tempeh, wheat free tamari, miso, and soy sauce.

32
Internal Pollution: the Glorious Universe Within

Have you taken out the garbage lately? If not, where are you storing it? As an innocent freckle-faced child of the 50's, I recall sprawling on my twin bed on a sunny day watching gossamer particles float aimlessly through sunbeams. As soon as the sunbeams left, the microscopic particles disappeared, but they were still there. "Am I inhaling this and if so, what is it, where does it come from, and where's it going?"

We scour our homes, wash clothes, and change the car oil filter, and in the AM, shave, wash hands, brush and floss teeth, get neatly dressed and comb our hair. How often do you clean out the inside of your car or house? What about changing the furnace filter every three months? Since Sandi and I live downtown the air is a stew of industrial snark. After observing the accumulated filter filth, I realized my loving family, too, is inhaling caustic waste by-products that cannot be seen by the naked eye. The furnace filter was gross. Since these particles are almost invisible as they float through the air, where do they go after entering our lungs? The universe created our Holy Temple with self-cleansing mechanisms: our skin, lymph nodes, our elimination system, and the blood-filtering liver, which has the biggest responsibility. But in today's chemically saturated society, America's gizzards are overwhelmed, especially with pharmaceuticals. Your internal "Kno-Zone" blocks energy / Chi flow throughout the Holy Temple, leaving you less than whole. Walking down the street we inescapably inhale air saturated with industrial chemicals and Chem Trails.

The average American carries 6-8 pounds of accumulated toxins from the environment, including factory food, household cleaners, antibiotics, chem-trails, growth hormones, estrogen, herbicides, preservatives, artificial sweeteners and flavors, food colorings, soot, dishwashing detergent, toxic laundry detergent, heavy metals, high fructose corn syrup, pop stars of this nefarious farce we call a food system.

Synthetic children's vitamins   overflow with toxic sweeteners and chemical colorings which can cause violent, aberrant behavior. Red dye 40 is exceptionally sinister. Household cleaners such as Lemon Pledge, give off toxic fumes we breathe as well. OTC medications dominate the list. Caveat emptor.

Greed-driven U.S. industry knuckle draggers manufacture 6 trillion pounds a year of 9,000 different chemicals and without a shred of guilt, and year after year, dump billions of microscopic pounds of industrial chemicals into our sacred air and water. The Fitzgerald Report reports, as of 1998, there were over 75,500 synthetic chemicals in processed food consumer products, industry and agriculture. Toxic body symptoms were: fatigue, headaches, muscle aches, right shoulder pain, poor appetite, heart burn, nausea, irritability, depression, PMS, menopausal symptoms, infertility, cancer, endometriosis, prostate problems, skin rashes, allergies, weak immunity, addictions, fungus and parasites. We apply chemicals to our skin, hair, underarms, teeth and nails to clean, moisturize and polish, protect from the sun, or to smell nice. If you put it on your skin, you're drinking it in. Internal pollution can cause your allergies, diverticulitis, and a delightful assortment of GI ails incubating in the dark recesses of your colon.

Research clearly proves that our bodies aren't capable of purging today's constellation of toxins and chemicals we inhale or ingest daily. They simply accumulate in our cells (especially fat cells), tissues, blood, organs, colon, and liver and remain stored for an indefinite length of time, causing all kinds health mayhem. If we feed our Holy Temple high quality, chemical free, living, local and nutritious whole foods it protects the Temple-the home of our wandering soul energy. Consider cleaning out your innards where who we are resides. We are a narcissistic, materialistic, consumer-driven society that seems to only care how the outside of our body and car appear to judgmental peers. "I've got leaky gut syndrome, anal seepage and I'm miserable, but my skin sure looks terrific."

The normal overweight person carries 10 meals with them in their gut. It's simple: there's no fiber in red meat and potatoes, whiskey, beer, and pie. A colonoscopy is not cleansing enough, but it's a brave start. A colonic restores, rebalances, and refreshes our hard-working colons. A bi-annual colonic is a good way to get rid of food that's been hanging around too long rotting at 98.6°. When you receive a colonic, the 99 degree water goes up inside and then flushes out almost 15 times to be sure to clean out all the crevices and convolutions where the food and hubba-bubba you ate when you were six is still dawdling.

Be sure to drink a probiotic beverage like Kombucha, and water after a cleanse to re-supply the good bacterial flora; do the same after any antibiotic treatment has exited your system. Exercise sufficiently. Whatever exercise you perform will encourage your Temple to sweat and excrete many toxins. Toxic? You might be if you suffer from frequent fatigue, low energy, flatulence, gas and bloating, excess weight food allergies, impaired digestion, irritability, mood swings, bad breath, recurring headaches, chronic constipation, irritable bowel syndrome, pooch belly, food cravings, metallic taste in mouth, hemorrhoids and Candida infection.

Before you begin, please visit your local allopathic, integrative or naturopathic physician. Start your healthy lifestyle first before you detox, so you have a reserve to allow your liver to do its job properly. Failing to do this overwhelms the liver's ability to process substances being eliminated, and you could become very sick. Exercise some down-home common sense. Your Creator will be pleased.

33
Get "Real" Patriotic with Food

Let the dietary Renaissance begin! Finally, the first governmental admission the red, white, and blue American diet is, one bite at a time, making us chronically ill and chubby, eroding the foundation of a once great nation.

For decades it's been going in one ear and out the other, but our U.S. Army, who historically marches on its stomach, recently determined creating quality recruits starts at the chow line with real, honest-to-goodness, genuine food. They're presently training soldiers to make healthier, fresher food choices, since the foods soldiers were taught to eat the last eight decades sabotaged their health, thereby inhibiting them from being the best they could be. This, too, applies to the esprit de corp and health of aging veterans throughout life's tour of duty.

What's placed into the Temple affects everything significant to American society: health, happiness, employment, productivity, education, the economy, and freedom. Fueled by a fixed diet of industrial rubbish, more turn to violent crime, bullying runs amok and good folks are defenseless to health skirmishes. Fox-holed with disease rates, education and fitness failures, and morally unacceptable health care costs bankrupting families, America's life, liberty and the pursuit of happiness plummets.

Standard, meat-heavy American food fare lacks fiber and bogs down digestion causing constipation and flatulence that impedes bowel evacuation. Foods like gluten, dairy and corn lead to allergies and ignite fire-fights of flatulence. Toxic compounds entering your Temple through factory feedlot animal husbandry and devitalized, processed grains hinder weight loss, and increase the foe of inflammation, the cause of 70 percent of America's diseases. Today, supermarket, corn-fed meats, farm raised salmon, and grocery sushi are treated with carbon monoxide. Not your grandpa's happy, grass-fed cattle. When the Temple can't purge toxic waste through bowel movements, it rids rotting food and toxins through stinky pits and foul breath.

Courageous U.S. troops are saying hello to fresh produce, granola, yogurt, beans, whole grains, guacamole and salsa and saying "hasta la vista, baby" to unctuous biscuits and sausage gravy, cheese burgers with fries, white bread, and sugary beverages, gurgling through their veins and arteries. While these foods titillate taste buds, they are IED's to intellectual, spiritual, and physical health. In America 5,000 die and 350,000 citizens become hospitalized, causalities of the American diet of, well, death. A diet allied to rapid aging, cancer, heart disease, Alzheimer's, obesity and diabetes, leaving troupes defenseless to invading disease. In the 20-year CARDIA study, researcher's tracked habits of 5,000 healthy adults living in four American cities and found everyday fast-food consumption was directly associated with changes in body weight and insulin resistance, a warning sign for type 2 diabetes. You might feel stimulated after sugary, fat-laden, fast-food breakfasts, but when your blood sugar crashes later, both your brain and your body will have trouble marching in step. American seniors suffer too many sick days wasting away in bed, an inability to focus, failure to learn, and lack creativity. More than an inactive lifestyle, smoking, and consuming booze, processed and canned foods are un-friendly interlopers to human health.

Clearly, no one deserves being attacked by the low-grade foods we're aggressively encouraged to devour. If patriotic Americans don't speak up and demand immediate, honest changes to predatory Big Foods lack of scruples and fraudulent food propaganda, we won't survive. America will fall, brought down by information terrorists: the consequences of a malnourished, chronically diseased population. It's not easy shifting hard-wired eating traditions. The University Of Minnesota School Of Public Health says the typical American meal preys on man's primordial fondness for fatty, grilled meats, bad fats, salts, and toxic sugar. BTW: Did you know sugar fertilizes cancer cells? CBS did a report exposing that Cancer cells adore high fructose corn syrup the most.

A friend with serious heart disease, a battle of the bulge, and no colon due to cancer, still opts to eat, "...by golly, what I dam well please. I fought in two wars so I could have free choice." In these battle-worn cases, wave the white flag then love them with all your heart, because you cannot change the feeble mind-set of, "You gotta die from somethin'." Get real, put on your big boy pants, and be part of the joyous solution.

34
Change: a Necessary Evil

"How dare you propose I stop eating the way my parents taught me? If it was good enough for them, by-golly, it's good enough for me." As the kids today articulate, that's "lamo."

Accepting man's imperfect humanness, everyone struggles letting go of comforting family rituals, stepping outside their dietary comfort zone. At the grocery, folks instinctively reach for expedient sources of food. Ergo, for their daily 3-squares, Americans suckle on the teats of Big Food, not honest, home cookin' where love is the most vital ingredient. As a result, we've become a sickly bunch due to the proliferation of abnormal man-made substances our cells can't utilize to sustain a healthy Holy Temple. The more fresh food gets altered, the sicker a nation becomes. If we are not healthy, we're not happy. If we're not healthy, we're powerless to contribute to the betterment of society. When we're not healthy, we exhibit disrespect for the Holy Temple, the only real home we have in this life.

Change is allegedly constant. But, we like things just the way they are, thank you. Strangely enough, we vainly change our fashion styles, hair, make-up and our cars, but give precious little thought to modifying the un-holy dietary assault on the Temple inner ecology with dead, albeit convenient food. "I've lived this long, why should I change now?" At 90, small dietary changes open up a big ol' can of "feel good." Living is breathtakingly sacred. Why would anyone, for the sake of flavor and instant gratification, compromise their self-worth, especially when every moment counts? Show yourself some love.

Before the Industrial Revolution, American communities bartered, shared and canned fresh food, constructing supportive, peaceful communities centered on local family farms bursting with sustainable sun-blessed produce -- when dairy farmers, bee keepers, and livestock farmers fed their stock a celestially ordained diet. One-hundred years ago everyone knew local farmers by their first name, shaking their calloused milking hand as they greeted. An ecologically centered community knits itself together with threads of peace, friendship, and the sharing of fresh, home-made foods simmered with love.

Grandma would have a conniption if she knew folks today eat laboratory-altered food fare shipped from a factory 2,000 carbon footprint miles away. Next time you grocery shop, scrutinize the shelves creaking from the burden of faux foods and then ask yourself, "Did these foods exist 100 years ago?" Big Food cons and flimflammers get satisfaction from suckering you into buying their products, so they use emotion, bright colors on the packages, inviting photos of the products and make dubious nutritional or health claims on the label. Yes, they're appealingly retailed, but are you really looking at them for what they truly are, or have you become robotically habituated to Pillsbury and Uncle Ben? We become comfortably numb with the grocery environment and don't take kindly to change. It freaks folks out and makes them uncomfortably angry, forcing them to examine something they normally don't wish to consider: the purity, sanctity, and source of food and its overall effects on the Temple.

We've witnessed mind-blowing changes in our eating habits during our numerous trips around the sun, and I'm beginning to believe many of these changes are causing the wheels to come off our cherished American way of life. Nothing has changed more than America's farming procedures, food production methods, and the grocery store experience. Even though we know a certain food damages our Temple, curiously, it seems to be the new norm, and folks demonstrate no compunction, consuming unhealthy, pre-made foods. Instead, they brag. For the first time in man's history, we will soon need to learn how to eat and cook all over again. Shipping food all over the country and world will become too expensive, leaving communities to procure local products only and cook with the seasons like our ancestors.

Remember the family-bonding, joyous act of cooking from scratch with fresh, local ingredients? Familiarity may or may not breed contempt, but it certainly breeds comfort. Change doesn't always have to be bad. Change for the better is good. Change in the way we eat causes changes in others.

35
Not So "Cool" Whip

Delivering my *Eat Right Now* program at a local hospital, a frail gal with an oxygen mask covering her mouth and nose approached my podium with her rolling, squeaking tank of oxygen in tow. "Is Cool Whip bad for me?" she whispered.

"How much do you eat, dear?" I asked, "Oh, 'bout a tub a day," she faintly responded, "I love it." You could have knocked me over with a Poop Tart as I explained "Cruel Whip" contains manmade ingredients that lead to heart disease, obesity, cancer, diabetes, and a build-up of toxins. Cool Whip is imitation: full of air, so you're eating mostly water and air for twice what it would cost to whip real cream. If you have heart disease, eating Cruel Whip is a subconscious death wish. Love yourself a bit more, okay?

Cruel Whip technology was invented by William A. Mitchell, an ethically damaged food douchebag at General Foods. The key to the technology was the creation of a whipped cream-like product that could be distributed in a frozen state from grocery chains and kept in the refrigerator. Wired Magazine reports the ingredients are real humdingers. Cool Whip contains hydrogenated coconut and palm oil, which when left unprocessed, are good for the heart, but the process of hydrogenation abnormally alters their cosmic structure. Trans-fats are officially banned in major cities all over the U.S. because of their direct link to heart disease.

Another disgraceful ingredient is high fructose corn syrup (HFCS). UCLA researchers have revealed cancer cells love it. In lab tests, pancreatic cancer cells quickly fed on the corn refiner's claptrap and used it to divide and proliferate rapidly within the Holy Temple. Another study conducted by Duke University researchers, once again implicated high-fructose corn syrup in a heightened risk of liver damage. A diet high in HFCS makes lab rats fatter than other diets. By the way, HFCS is found in nearly all processed foods. Smell what I'm cooking?

Not sure about you, but I'm crazy about Polysorbate 60, a precursor to anti-freeze and the lubricant used in prophylactics. You heard me correctly: rubbers. This gives Cool Whip it's creamy, fatty "mouth-feel." I'm not convinced this is what our Creator intended us to place into our Holy Temple. As my grandkids would say, "euwww."

Next, the Jerkonians who need our love add a scrumptious blob of sorbitan monostearate, a synthetic wax sometimes used as a, yep, hemorrhoid cream. This unholy substance is used to keep it from turning liquid. Next, they gently stir in xanthan and guar gums, natural thickeners which retard the formation of ice crystals, preserving its seductive deceiving fluffiness. You can wrap dog-doo in pretty paper, but it's still doggie-doo. Have no fear, Chef Wendell is here! May I suggest a simple substitute? Sandi takes a container of organic yogurt, plops it into a fine mesh strainer lined with cheesecloth or tea towel, and lets it drain overnight, resting over a vessel to catch the liquid whey. Coconut milk yogurt is the best. What's left is a thick and creamy, full flavored topping. Don't discard the liquid whey. Drink it down in a smoothie, since it's loaded with B-vitamins and protein. Waste not, want not.

The human Holy Temple works best when its fuel is genuine, not concocted by laboratory full of giddy chef-wannabes. If you must, use whipping cream, but make it a rare treat, not a daily ritual. I don't care if you have carpal tunnel, real cream in moderation is the lesser of two evils. Dust off the ol' wire whisk for goodness sakes and then occasionally switch hands.

Your heavenly gift of a Temple is the only true home you have. Be a responsible steward, respect yourself, and defend your loving family from the relentless, all-out assault on human health by Big Food, FDA, USDA dietary terrorists. Sadly, the money grubbers couldn't possibly care less about your health, but I honestly do.

36
Children's Lunches

Rearing a healthy, happy child is a privilege. Training children as they mature and grow can be joyous; swaying children towards obesity and diabetes is heartbreaking and irresponsible.

Recently, during one of my lectures, an adorable group of schoolchildren shared family eating customs. One girl ate 4 cookies and drank flavored chocolate milk. Another ran late so Mommy gave her a candy bar and Mt. Dew. Later she defended, "I normally eat better. Today, Mommy was running late, so she didn't have time to toast my "Pop Tart." ("Poop Tarts.") They ate 'em at my age. Mommy says, "If it's good enough for her, good enough for me." OMG! Some parents get overly stressed around "healthy" foods. It seems some parents have issues with taking time to cook healthy meals. Most parents do a great job; some not as well as they should.

America adores tradition, but has difficulty letting go. What happens when parents suddenly discover their beloved eating traditions deteriorate childhood health? For example: The American Institute for Cancer Research announced habitually eating processed meats, hot dogs, bacon and bologna, increase risk of cancer, yet we worship smoked meats. I've been called un-American for bashing the toxic icons. Or, how artificial food coloring and flavoring in Fruit Loops and fruit drinks worsens ADHD, causes hyperactivity, aggressive and violent behavior? Finally, will loving parents heed the *Journal of Pediatrics* report stating Vitamin D-3 deficiency is so widespread it poses a huge threat to the future health of an entire generation?

We learn early in life, food, sleep and air are essential to earthling's survival. Maturing bodies require 40 essential vitamins and 90 minerals a day from fresh, whole foods to protect and provide the tools needed to develop normally.

What kids eat today and until they are 18 sets the blueprint for their future mental and physical health. Because no one could intake enough food to achieve that total, a food-based, multi-vitamin is requisite. The quality of their daily diet instantly becomes important, considering the reports stating this will be the first generation of children whose parents will outlive their parents due to nutritional illiteracy and malnourishment. Besides breathing, eating is one of the most important actions we perform for survival. Even kids can acquire health problems like cancer, heart disease, asthma, muscular dystrophy and more. Purity, variety and balance are infinitely essential.

To lovingly encourage children to eat well, parents can set the model by eating wholesome foods themselves. Otherwise, children will learn from other peers. Considering the cost of healthcare, tradition can be an occasional treat, not a daily custom.

37
Inflammation: 21st Century's Silent Killer

Grossly erroneous, the medical fraternity recklessly teaches Americans to vilify cholesterol. Did you know brains and cells are totally dependent upon abundant supplies of cholesterol? Cholesterol has long been seen as the key culprit in cardiovascular disease. However, half of all heart attacks occur in people with normal cholesterol levels, which suggest another factor is at work.

Research indicates cholesterol's role as partner in crime to inflammation: the flood of white blood cells and chemicals our immune system unleashes to ward off damage or infection, the true cause of cardiovascular disease. The fire comes from many unexpected places. Inflammation is the Holy Temple's immediate first-aid reaction to soothe and heal itself from damage caused by a virus, gluten, corn, soy, and dairy allergies, bacteria, fungus, environmental toxins, fake foods, or an injury. It appears what we don't know about inflammation is causing many chronic diseases, while authorities set back and watch. Bad karma! What happened to the Hippocratic Oath, "First, do no harm?"

"Inflammation is the common denominator in nearly all of the diseases we deal with," says James O'Keefe, MD, director of preventive cardiology at the Mid America Heart Institute in Kansas City, Missouri. "Heart disease, diabetes, dementia -- they're all tied to inappropriate, low-grade, chronic inflammation." Visualize the inflammation process as a light bulb. When left on constantly, the bulb burns out faster than if it's turned off during non-use. When the inflammation fails to turn off, the immune system becomes compromised due to overwork and overuse. Once the protective immune system is compromised, all forms of nasty chronic disease occur, but not just inflammatory diseases. We're talking cancer, fibromyalgia, heart disease and stroke, obesity, Alzheimer's, Parkinson's, MS, and Lupus. Internal inflammation is often caused by bacterial infection, but can also be caused by disorders such as allergies, anemia, arthritis, asthma, autoimmune diseases, Crohn's disease, osteoarthritis, peptic ulcer disease, or ulcerative colitis.

Studies show a substance known as C-reactive protein (CRP), one of the so-called markers released by cells during the inflammation
process, may be more effective than cholesterol in calculating your risk of heart attack and cardiovascular events. To test for chronic inflammation, politely request your family physician to order a C-reactive protein evaluation. Chronic inflammation is normally seen in good folks who have diets with an unbalanced ratio of Omega-6 to Omega-3 EFA's. Omega-3 EFA's soothe internal inflammation, thus kicking chronic disease in the tushy. The DOA American diet woefully lacks Omega-3 from healthy sources of fish oil, wild-caught fish, nuts and flax and chia seeds. Due to our highly-processed American diet laden with dreadful hydrogenated oils, folks get more much more 6 than 3. An ideal balance is a one-to-one ratio of Omega-6 to 3's. With America's emphasis on vegetable cooking oils high in Omega-6 oils, most folks get a ratio of about 26:1 rather than 1:1. Bread, bagels, potato chips, cookies, cakes, candy bars, most prepared foods from the supermarket, hamburgers, pizza, other fast food and most restaurant meals all contain too much Omega 6.

Some Omega 6 fats are essential. The problem is junk-food addicted Americans eat way too much Omega 6. When you have a choice, eat fresh unprocessed living foods. Pick virgin olive oil, unrefined coconut oil over peanut, safflower, or Wesson-type oils, and use in moderation. Grass-fed organic butter is very low in Omega 6; margarine and vegetable oils are high. Grass-fed meats actually lower bad cholesterol levels. Alas, most grocery red meats are fed GMO corn, other dead cow parts, antibiotics, insecticides, growth hormones, and, well you get the unholy picture. No need for alarm. You haven't done anything wrong. You don't intentionally eat foods to get disease; you eat them because everyone else does. Stand up, take a stance, and eat from the local universal farm-acy, not a food factory. Debauched Big Food misled a trusting patriotic nation for 100 years for profit. To them, wholesome human nutrition is a joke and innocents agonize. It's only about flavor, money and addiction. Not the greater good. No different than a street corner drug dealer.

38
Soy has an Evil Twin

Years back, I studied Ayurveda. In this ancient medical model, diet and efficient digestion are the foundation of your mental, physical, and spiritual destiny. Without proper, cosmic nutrition, a connection with our higher source cannot be achieved and meditation becomes ineffective.

It was part of my job to cook a daily fresh meal for the staff of a Holistic Hospital. I prepared a kitchari that day with sautéed zucchini, turmeric, edamame, ginger and garlic. Assuming, as we all do, I was okay with soy beans, I added Edamame to the dish for some clean protein. I thought. As a visiting Ayurvedic priest quietly and consciously ate his food with gratitude, he slowly turned his head, looked me in the eyes and said, "Soy is slow suicide," gesturing with his fork at the soy beans, and went back to mindfully chewing his food.

In Ayurveda, foods we ingest are divided into three categories: poison, medicine, or neutral. Poison is defined as anything that hinders digestion. Medicine is considered to be anything that we ingest that aids the digestive process. Neutral is anything we ingest that gives support and nourishment without either aiding or hindering the digestive process. It's all about efficient digestion.

Kitchari, a recipe you'll find in the following recipes, is unique because it falls under both the neutral and medicinal categories. It not only provides nourishment for the Holy Temple but, due to its spice combination, benefits digestion. This makes kitchari an ideal food of choice during times of stress on the body, during an illness, periods of overwork, or change of seasons. It's also especially groovy to use glorious fresh, living, fibrous food as part of an internal cleansing regime.

As evidence on the toxicity of soy isoflavones accumulates, warnings have begun to appear in the popular press. An article appearing in the *Washington Post* Health Section was entitled: "You have to be soy careful: tofu and similar foods may be beneficial, but some experts fear that too much could be unsafe." Writing for the *New York Times*, health columnist Marian Burros published the following comment on isoflavone supplements, which provide 50-100 mg isoflavones per capsule: "Against the backdrop of widespread praise there is growing suspicion soy, despite its touted benefits, may pose some health hazards. Not one of the eighteen scientists interviewed was willing to say taking isoflavones was risk free." Caveat Emptor.

39
Comfort Food; an Oxymoron

Comfort foods are our best friends. They abidingly put forward generous bowls of "feel-good." Familiarity may or may not breed contempt, but it definitely breeds comfort.

We repeatedly change hair styles, makeup, clothing fashion, our cars and their oil, but when it comes to changing ones perspective of what shapes the condition of one's mind, soul and body, most folks flee in terror, ignoring harmful health outcomes to the Temple. We've yet to link food with disease. To most, it's merely ephemeral amusement.

Do you eat white bread and bologna? If so, consider rats won't eat white bread in laboratory conditions and according to the American Cancer Society, bologna, as American as apple pie, is an identified carcinogen. Grilled cheese on white bread with Kraft industrial "cheese" singles and butter is mighty tasty, but a notorious delivery system for artery plaque. White bread is stripped of cosmic nutrients during ruthless processing. That's why they fortify the "catfish bait" with useless synthetic vitamins. This high glycemic crap-olo makes you temporarily feel groovy, but spikes glucose, ergo aggravating the pancreas and sets the stage for 'diabesity.' Substitute whole grain Ezekiel, gluten-free, and Rudi's bakery breads, grass-fed organic butter, Earth Balance or similar Omega-3 margarine, and rice or almond cheese slices for a grandkid-approved grilled cheese, full of protein and colon-protecting fiber.

"Eek! There's a scam in my soup!" Campbell's Healthy Request and low sodium tomato soups contain the identical bogus nutrients, cancerous BPA, salt, sugar, and sodium as regular tomato soups, but cost more since consumers will pay the price for a familiar product perceived as healthy. Both low sodium and normal tomato contain 1.5 grams of fat, while regular has 0 grams of fat. Big friggin' deal. Don't be easy marks; seek Pacific Natural Foods soups in a box in the health section, or make a big batch and freeze the excess.

Addicted to oily french fries, corn or potato chips? If you dig lubricating your innards three-in-one style, go ahead, it's a free country. Baked potato with butter, bacon, and sour cream is a stent-cardiologist dream, so seriously, try baked sweet potatoes, drizzled with real maple syrup, Stevia, or honey. A plain baked potato with Greek yogurt, salsa or mashed taters with almond milk, garlic, and olive oil are equally comforting. Toss in a handful of fibrous ground flax or a chia seed for accelerated peristalsis which gives pesky toxins the heave-ho.

Do you have a weakness for boxed, extruded crackers or cheese curls loaded with artificial cheese, MSG, GMO corn oil and sumptuous chemical flavoring? Change to toasted whole wheat bread sticks, black bean chips, rice chips, Wheat Thins, low-fat potato chips, whole wheat pita bread, baked corn chips, or pretzels. All box stores carry healthy versions of your beloved crunchy friends.

While traveling and giving lectures, all I'm offered are pitchers of Half & Half or petite vessels of angioplasty-flavored creamers. Powdered cream, the Anti-Christ of them all, may taste delicious, but toss them out for the respect of the Temple. Try almond or coconut milk.

Bless Uncle Ben's heart. When he "perverted" rice, the processing stripped the once nourishing whole grain of its fiber and heavenly nutrients. No wonder so many have diabetes. Walk on the wild side and change from white rice to brown rice or quinoa. After that, change from white flour pasta and opt for Barilla Plus Pasta with whole grains, bean flour pasta, barley, lentils, Omega 3, fiber and protein. Little changes in the way you eat will cause good changes in others. We're all happy when we're healthy.

40
Vegaphiobia

Until I was 40, I ate against my cosmic nature. When I began eating more fruits and veggies from the universal apothecary and less processed rubbish, amazing skills surfaced I did not know existed. By not feeding myself the proper diet designed for humans, I discovered I was blunting my innate skills and my true self, too. Fruits and vegetables are a natural source of energy and give the body the building blocks to keep going.

I sometimes wonder if the mass confusion, conflicting headlines, disinformation terrorists, and such are by design. No, *really*, I'm not a conspiracy theorist, but mind you, it is highly profitable to keep people fat, and sick, and coming back for more help, isn't it?

I can't imagine why America has never been encouraged to eat what our Creator originally designed. Instead, our health is in the hands of advertisers, greedy-to-the-bone bankers, and biased commodities brokers. But the reality is, advertising exerts a mighty influence over what we choose to eat and feed our families. If your children watch television, watch it with them and discuss the cunning advertising. Also discuss ads in magazines, newspapers, and billboards as well on the internet and on in-school advertising. Talk about what the ads are trying to sell and how to know if what they say is true. Observe your children's reactions. Children don't like to be tricked any more than adults.

No one was born to hate vegetables, they were taught. Despite all the campaigns to promote fruit and vegetable intake, only a third of Americans eat two or more pieces of fruit per day and 25 percent don't eat any vegetables at all. Sigh... And, why not? Recent research shows the five common reasons for not eating healthy: availability, cost, nutritional illiteracy, confusion, biased advertising semantics, time constraints, and taste. The National Cancer Institute recommends five to nine ½ cup servings of fresh, local fruits and vegetables per day to ward off cancer and other diseases. Unfortunately, only about a quarter of adults do, even though it's fairly easy and the natural thing to do. Say hello to a farmer's market.

Almost everyone needs to eat more fruits and vegetables. A growing body of research shows fruits and vegetables are critical to upholding good health. To get the amount that's recommended, most people need to increase the amount of raw fruits and vegetables they currently eat every day. Uncooked vegetables and fruits contain substances called "phytonutrients." These are compounds that help the plant fight off disease. They are powerful defenders of our own health, too, fighting chronic diseases like cancer, heart disease, and blood pressure. Fruits and vegetables contain essential vitamins, minerals, and fiber which help protect your Holy Temple from chronic diseases. Compared with people who consume a diet with only small amounts of fruits and vegetables, those who eat more generous amounts as part of a healthful diet are likely to have reduced risk of chronic diseases, including stroke, and perhaps, other cardiovascular diseases, and certain cancers.

- Pre-cut vegetables into serving-size portions and place in the refrigerator for easy access. Make your vegetables as convenient to eat as any other snack food, and you *will* eat more of them.

- Create a salad bar with healthy dips and those vegetable decorations you learned to make. Dips include low fat salad dressing, peanut butter, cottage cheese, and salsa.
- With renal disease and kidney disorders, eating fruit and vegetables, or drinking orange juice, with iron-rich foods is a good idea.
- When serving hamburgers, sloppy joes, pizza or any other kid-pleasing fare, toss in some shredded carrots or broccoli. Just a small amount will blend right into a red sauce and boost the nutritional value.
- Try grilled kabobs. Cut bite-sized pieces of vegetables and grill them on skewers, or alternate with chunks of meat. Add a tasty marinade.

41
Consequences

Addicted to fast food? You're not alone. Here's an accounting of some of the charming consequences of worshiping dead food:

Personal health: This diet causes rapid aging and the aggressive development of degenerative disease: Cancer, heart disease, diabetes, obesity, Alzheimer's disease, etc. The population also remains highly susceptible to infectious disease.

Health care costs: In a nation that follows a bad diet, health care costs spiral out of control, eventually consuming a quarter (or more) of the GDP, driving the nation into bankruptcy.

Education: Growing up on this bad diet, children suffer severe cognitive impairment and are unable to learn in school. In time, academic achievement of the nation falls sharply, and the great "dumbing down" of the population accelerates.

Employment and economy: A sick, diseased population is very expensive to maintain on the payrolls of Corporate America. Poisoned by processed food diets, workers suffer from repeated sick days and poor cognitive performance at work (inability to focus, failure to learn, failure to create new ideas, etc.), all of which make the workforce increasingly expensive for corporations to maintain. Not surprisingly, this causes yet a further shift of jobs to other nations where workers are more productive, healthier and less expensive.

Violent crime: With their brains fueled by junk foods (and with failed education giving them few options for earning an honest living), more people turn to crime. In time, the prisons become filled with people incarcerated for behavior that could have been at least partially prevented with proper nutrition.

Happiness: With disease rates skyrocketing, violent crime on the rise, education failures rampant and health care costs bankrupting families, happiness plummets to all-time lows.

Genetic integrity: As junk food consumption continues through multiple generations, the *genetic integrity* of the population erodes. Birth defects increase while fertility rates plummet. The population increasingly becomes haunted with unhealthy genetic mutations that promote yet more disease in future generations.

Economic productivity: Poor nutrition leads to disastrous economic productivity. Powered by junk foods, the population becomes virtually useless as a workforce. Instead of producing new ideas, new products and new innovations that improve the world, people wallow around like Yabba the Hut, mindlessly eating Fritos while watching YouTube. As economic productivity plummets, employers shift jobs to overseas markets where people often demonstrate much higher levels of productivity.

World Leadership: With its population falling behind the world academically and economically, the nation loses its leadership position on the world stage and begins to lose its leverage for maintaining the dominance of its currency.

Democracy & Freedom: When the voters subsist on a dead diet, their minds are clouded and child-like. They are easily manipulated to vote for politicians who are essentially "entertainers" who look good on TV, but have no real ability to improve the long-term situation for the country. Voters under the influence and addiction to junk foods, elect the very people who continue to herd the nation off the cliff of disease and disaster. Wake up!

42
The Secret Life of Milk

Like clockwork, twice weekly the Roberts milk truck rumbled through our 50's east side neighborhood. Before America became litigiously trigger happy, the friendly driver in his white starched uniform and hat would thrill me by letting me hitch hike along for a few streets before he'd tell me to skedaddle. What a happy memory. Good ol' wholesome milk from a lactating bovine pumped full of delicious Rbgh growth hormones.

Iconic milk represents purity, wholesomeness, and all things good. So when did milk get to be so essential to the survival of our species? When corporations learned cow milk was profitable, advertising executives went to work brainwashing every American that unless they put milk in their tea or coffee, cakes, puddings, or chicken gravy, they were downright un-American. Well, America fell into a well-crafted marketing program designed to make the citizenry dependent on milk, America's beverage. Today's milk is a far cry from what our ancestors drank. BTW: Did you know man is the only species on earth that drinks milk from another lactating species?

If I were a grass-eatin' milk cow, I'd be concerned about the source of my next pay check. Actually, milk cows are worried about a lot more serious issues such as growth hormones, rGBH, infected teat (PUS) residue, chicken droppings, cow parts and corn in their food, anti-biotics, and their living accommodations. You have a birthright to avoid these compounds. The Great Creator made them grass-eating, ruminant vegetarians for crying out loud, and man feeds them the last thing they should eat: GMO corn. Again, even the most greedy, rich, intelligent and blindly arrogant man cannot improve on the works of our Creator. Send them some love.

Want pus with your cookies? If you down a glass of cow's milk, you will, according to the *New York Times*. The dairy industry knows there's a problem with pus (white blood cells) in milk caused by ultra-aggressive milking. Infection sets in, and the luscious white blood cells leach into the milk. Factory dairy farmers try to control the rampant mastitis with large doses of antibiotics that wind up in the milk. Children are particularly vulnerable to the effects of too many antibiotics, which researchers believe can inhibit the development of the immune system. The chocolate covers up the bitter taste of greed.

Everyone has seen the milk commercials with celebrities sporting white milk mustaches. PETA has their version that asks, "Got PUS." Factory farms milk the cows so aggressively and demand so much milk that the dairy cows get infections on their teats. There is discussion in Washington now on how much pus the American public can tolerate with this sad and pitiable human behavior? Support your local dairy.

Milk and milk products have played an important role in America's history since 1611, when the first dairy cows were moved to Jamestown, Virginia. Since those early days, the industry has continued to serve the nutritional needs of a growing nation with a wide selection of products.

Whoa! Let's back up the ol' milk wagon, chat and give the exhausted milkers a rest. One hundred years ago, milk production per cow was estimated at 1,700 quarts annually; today, the average has leaped to more than 8,200 quarts per cow. The liquid sold as milk in supermarkets bears little resemblance to milk produced by a well-treated, grass-fed, brown-eyed cow.

The Weston Price foundation claims pasteurized milk, "...is associated with allergies, increased tooth decay, colic in infants, mucus, growth problems in children, osteoporosis, arthritis, heart disease and cancer." Sally Fallon, president of the Weston A. Price Foundation, contends vegetarian cows peacefully grazed on pasture grass rather than jammed into pens and force-fed corn and other dead cows, will produce milk that is healthy and pathogen-free.

The U.S. has the highest rate of Crohn's ever recorded. Crohn's disease is a chronic debilitating inflammatory disease of the bowel with an increase in modern societies. Evidence has implicated a bacterium that is transmitted via pasteurized cow's milk in the etiology of this disease. A bacterium called Mycobacterium avium paratuberculosis (MAP) found in dairy products survives the heat of pasteurization and causes inflammatory bowel disease in a variety of animals, including monkeys and chimpanzees. In the last few years, this same bacterium has been detected in a large percentage of humans who have Crohn's disease. Michael Greger, M.D. tells us there is now growing clinical, epidemiological, immunological, experimental, and DNA evidence that cow pus / white blood cells is the cause of Crohn's in people who drink milk from infected cows. Since transmission of this bacteria is facilitated by its presence inside pus cells, American milk drinkers may be at particularly high risk since the US has the highest permitted upper limit of milk pus cell concentration in the world—almost twice the international standard of allowable pus. By U.S. federal law, Grade A milk is allowed to have over a drop of pus per glass of milk. What a "revoltin' development" you got US in to this time, FDA. Shall we call them the Fraud and Deception Administration?

Repeat after me: Our children, our children, remember our children. This adoration of money has gone too far. It is reprehensible to suck folks in with marketing, and then begin bastardizing the product with harmful, un-Godly additives. An American tradition sold to the highest bidder, like a skuzzy, common, street corner drug dealer. Great Creator of all life, bless and forgive these lost, dark souls.

Genetically modifying milk is playing God. There is a potential concern that small changes to the nutritional content might have effects on infant bowel function. Dr. Eric Brunner, an epidemiologist at University College, London, says, "Genetic modification might lead to unpredicted and harmful changes in the nutritional status of the food." Ya think?

Raw milk consumption is growing. Selling raw, un-pasteurized milk is illegal in many states and the District of Columbia, and family farmers are being arrested at gun point. Whether or not raw milk carries pathogens depends totally on the way the milk is produced, how the animals are fed, and the care that's taken to keep the milk clean during production. What did folks do before Pasteur? Again, man is the only species on earth that drinks milk from another species. Contemplate that, my milk-breath friends!

43
I'm Coo-Coo for Coconuts

A long time ago, when wisdom ruled, coconut oil was in just about everything you ate. What misfortune since today, malleable Americans robotically condemn coconut oil because they were "told" it was a saturated fat associated with blocked arteries. The truth is unrefined, raw coconut oil, a medium-chain fatty acid, does not negatively affect blood cholesterol, but actually protects against heart disease and a constellation of Western diseases.

What I consider most creepy, exploiting fear? Big Food Jerkonians intentionally urged a gullible population to embrace sinister hydrogenated vegetable oil, a.k.a. trans fats, and millions died unnecessarily from heart disease   Other than injecting lard or tallow into your veins, hydrogenated oils are the most health-damaging, vile, dietary oils created my man's self-serving attempts to upstage God. This illustrates how corrupt leadership and greed for the proliferation of degenerative disease and the inept health care system has taken part in trashing a patriotic nation's entitlement of good health. We are the innocent victims of their appalling decisions, fueled by the love of money. Sigh... being American does not guarantee longer years. In fact, the United States has dropped from 24th in the world for life expectancy in 1999 to 49th in 2010. Critics say our so-called, best-in-the-world, most costly health care is the primary cause.   Question authority why they shun prevention and watch them squirm uncomfortably.

Virgin, unrefined, raw coconut oil found in some groceries and all community health food stores, is one of earth's most amazing, healing gifts. Its delicious, medium-chain fatty acids are rapidly converted into energy rather than wiggly fat. Refined coconut oil, on the other hand, is unhealthy due to heat and processing.   Unlike processed grocery vegetable oils, coconut oil does not form harmful by-products when heated to normal cooking temperature.

Modern medical science has revealed veiled secrets regarding coconut oil's numerous medicinal applications. Where coconut is in abundance, in the South Pacific, natives enjoy remarkably good health, free from aches, pains and many degenerative diseases such as heart disease, cancer, diabetes and arthritis. Health benefits of creamy coconut oil include hair and skin care. I've used it as a shave cream and Sandi says my face looks like a baby's bottom, which I trust is flattering. The diverse oil can be used for stress relief, maintaining cholesterol levels, weight loss, increase immunity, pesky toe fungus, proper digestion and metabolism, relief from kidney problems, heart disease, high blood pressure, diabetes, HIV and cancer, dental care, and bone strength. Phew, the list is too long. This is all attributed to its lauric acid, capric acid, and caprylic acid and its antimicrobial, antioxidant, antifungal, antibacterial mojo. The only other source of lauric acids and medium-chain fatty acids in such concentrations is in sacred mother's milk. Rich and creamy coconut milk, the heavy cream of South Asia, is super nutritious and brims with fiber, vitamin C, folate, selenium, minerals and electrolytes.

Called "the tree of life," one-third of the planet's inhabitants depend on coconut oil and milk for food. If coconut oil is so good, why have we been instructed to obediently vilify it? Disinformation campaigns designed by the soy, canola and lard cartels. It is simple: love of money, politics, half-truths and deliberate misinformation. You see, according to Bruce Fife, author of "The Coconut Miracle," the soybean industry carefully orchestrated a 1980's smear campaign against the coconut oil industry to profit from the public's fear of saturated fats linked with heart disease, another reason to distrust the soy boys. Immature rubbish in view of The Weston Price Foundation saying "unfermented" soybean oil contributes to thyroid disorder, especially in women, promotes kidney stones, weakens the immune system, and contributes to food allergies and digestive intolerances. Estrogen-like compounds in soybean oil foods can lower sperm count, according to the Harvard School of Public Health at the 63rd Annual Meeting of the American Society for Reproductive Medicine. The report by Jorge Chavarro, MD, ScD, reinforces concerns that soy negatively affects male fertility and testosterone. Bummer! The bottom line, soy sucks and should be sidestepped like cow pies, with the exception of fermented soy products like miso, tempeh, soy sauce and natto.

Abandoning unhealthful lifestyles and reverting to real, natural foods helps reverse many Western diseases manifesting in our bodies through the highly refined, biased diet of our modern society. You can do it.

Virgin, Unrefined Coconut Oil's Mojo

- Reduces risk of arteriosclerosis and related illnesses
- Reduces risk of cancer and other degenerative conditions
- Helps prevent bacterial, viral, and fungal (including yeast) infections
- Supports immune functions
- Soothes and helps skin — our largest organ
- Helps prevent osteoporosis
- Helps control diabetes
- Promotes weight loss
- Supports healthy metabolic function
- Provides an immediate source of energy
- Nourishes hair and controls dandruff
- Supplies fewer calories than other fats
- Supplies important nutrients necessary for good health
- Improves digestion and nutrient absorption
- Is highly resistant to spoilage (long shelf life)

44
Be Your Heart's Valentine

Our heart, the wellspring from which our true nature is revealed, is the dwelling of intuition, love, creativity, wisdom, gratitude, and faith, qualities generally associated with the mind. We know deep in our heart, the ever-beating orb is entwined with influencing and being influenced by everything we do, say, see, and eat.

Do you show love and compassion to your life-blood pumping pal? Dr. Gregory Martin, Indiana State Health Commissioner, advised heart-clutching vegaphobic Hoosiers, "We have to take a fresh look at our comfortable habits and apply better wisdom."

Open up your heart to new foods and love your way toward a heart-healthy diet. Give your heart the daily gift of antioxidant blueberries, potent disease-fighting foods. The delightful, dark blue jewels sparkle with fiber and vitamin C, are available fresh and frozen year long. How about wild caught salmon? If it's not antibiotic laden farm-raised salmon, it contains clean protein packed with heart-healthy Omega-3 fatty acid. The American Heart Association advises eating salmon and other Omega-3 rich foods, like chia seed and walnuts, twice weekly.

Popeye and Olive Oil knew that spinach is a powerhouse. Its rich, dark color comes from the phytochemicals, vitamins, folate and iron that protect against heartbreaking situations. Don't even flirt with grocery spinach unless it's organic. Non-organic spinach is sprayed liberally with cancerous chemicals. Consistently eating a variety of fresh organic highly vibrational fruits and vegetables, legumes, whole grains, and grass-fed dairy products lovingly protect a hungry heart and minimizes chances of "the big one."

Limiting certain fats proven to be unhealthy is important. Of the types of fat, saturated factory farm animal fat, and trans fats/hydrogenated oils greatly increase risk of obesity and coronary artery disease. Major sources of inflammatory saturated fat include beef, pork, butter, cheese, milk, and palm oils, but not raw, unrefined, virgin coconut oil. Hydrogenated oils are banned in many major U.S. cities since they are worse than saturated fat since raise HDL and lower LDL. Snarky trans fats lurk within deep-fried fast foods, bakery products, packaged snack foods, margarines and crackers. Things are gradually improving, fortunately.

Want to trash your health, consume canola oil, a member of the mustard family. The Weston Price Foundation say 'Con'-ola, a hyped flim-flam developed in Canada, is bogus oil engineered from the rapeseed plant. Canola is an excellent insect repellent and machine lubricant according to the EPA. Canola is found to be poisonous for all living things, including humans. It's also used as fuel and a solution to brighten the colored pages of magazines. To its credit, the FDA has taken a stance to protect babies from the unknown risks of canola oil and prohibits the contrived medium from being used in infant formula. Ya think?

Canola oil from the Rapeseed plant, toxic to humans, is listed as an insect repellent and lubricant was the main ingredient in the mustard gas used as weapons in WW II and Dessert Storm. When canola was engineered, the toxic erucic acid is supposed to be filtered out.

The effects of canola oil have been tested on humans, but biased studies on lab rats and pigs have shown that the consumption of canola led to an excess of fat and cholesterol in the blood, as well as hypertension, degeneration of the heart, kidney, adrenals, and thyroid gland. What a shock, you've been misled...again. According to Livestrong.com, Canada paid the U.S. FDA $50 million to recognize canola oil as safe. Originally, canola oil was never meant for human consumption, but has been used as an insecticide and may affect trans-fatty acid levels. Caveat emptor.

Instead, show your heart love with extra virgin olive oil, walnut or grape seed oil, fish oil, flax and chia oils, raw unrefined organic coconut oil, and modest quantities of sunflower, sesame, safflower, peanut, and ghee. Cottonseed oil is the filthiest. Remember, never let any oil reach the smoking point; heat destroys the love and turns oil cancerous. Rarely mentioned, fat from grass-fed beef actually contains Omega 3 fatty acids that reduce plaque. Factory farm concentration camps feed the brown-eyed furry vegetarian bovines other dead cows, ugh, mouth-watering growth hormones, appetite stimulants, pesticides, fertilizers, herbicides, and everyone's beloved aflatoxins.

This unholy grocery meat should be avoided like the Black Plague. Other health-appropriate options include winter squash, oatmeal, Navy beans, cinnamon-an anti-inflammatory, and apples including the peel. Be aware, dark chocolate is a nutrient and calorie-rich food. A little is wonderful, a lot is not.

Next Valentine's Day have a dalliance with your heart. By tenderly embracing real, living foods intended by creation to restore, rebuild, and sustain the Temple, you engrave a love note onto your heart saying, "I care." Eating greasy, sugary, dead bar-coded food with no fresh produce or whole grains heaps contempt upon your monogamous Temple. So, what's it going to be, Valentine?

45
Hey Bully! Your Mood's in the Food

A distraught, middle-school mother mumbled, "When my children come home from school, you'd think they were raised by jackals. On weekends, I can control what they eat and they're normal kids who gripe about their homework but respect Bob and me. After they eat the crap served at school, they come home bitchy, vulgar and inattentive. They're also restless and have trouble sleeping."

This current swell in aberrant behavioral social disorders and "bullyism" of all ages is a perfect example of the disruption of human nature by the swelling accumulation of alien pollutants accumulating in our collective internal ecosystem. Contemporary industrialized diets may be causing behavioral disorders such as hyperactivity, aggressive behavior, autism and Attention Deficit Disorder (ADD) by altering the architecture and workings of our brilliant brains. Today, thousands of synthetic chemicals have the official okeydokey for use in the processed-food industry. Many are known to have delightful carcinogenic properties. All affect your mood as profoundly as a drug. For a list of chemicals used in food production and their delightful side effects on our birthright of health, go to: http://www.cspinet.org/nah/05_08/chem_cuisine.pdf

Truth in Publishing declares virtually all modern diseases are caused by "metabolic disruptors" found in everyday foods. According to the International Trade Commission, major factors contributing to the occurrence of disease include adverse responses to food additives and intolerances to fake foods.

Succulent nitrosamines are used to give deli and smoked meats an alluring reddish color so they don't look putridly gray. Clinical studies monitoring children consuming nitrosamines revealed a fourfold increase of brain tumors and a 700% increase in leukemia. According to Sourcewatch.org, the human immune system properly recognizes chemical additives as toxic foreign terrorists and fights hard to expel them from the Temple. This strenuous act causes accelerated aging and ruthless biochemical reactions which place colossal stress on the immune system.

In a study of 27 British children, doctors at the Royal Prince Alfred Hospital concluded the preservatives in food caused irritability, antisocial behavior, inattention and sleep disturbance. When the doctors minimized the concentrations added to processed foods, the children's behavior improved significantly. In 2002, under double-blind, placebo-controlled tests at Aylesbury Jail, the British *Journal of Psychiatry* found nutritional supplements have a major impact on violent behaviors. The British prison trial showed when young men there were fed multivitamins, minerals and essential fatty acids 3, 6, 9, and junk food was prohibited, the number of violent offenses committed in the prison fell by 37 per cent.

Shun foods containing these shocking ingredients:
- Carbon monoxide - used to preserve color in grocery beef, salmon, tuna, turkey, pork and pre-made grocery sushi
- Sodium nitrite - in hot dogs, bacon, bologna, smoked fish and jerky
- MSG - used in soups, snacks, and some Chinese foods
- Aspartame/Nutra-Sweet - used to sweeten diet soda and gum
- Splenda and Sweet n' Low
- Yeast extract - in snacks
- Hydrogenated oils / trans fats
- High fructose corn syrup in virtually everything
- Saccharin
- Caffeine
- Olestra (snack foods)
- Acesulfame Kd in diet soda
- Artificial coloring and flavoring

- AP flour

Opt for real food that empowers the Holy Temple to do what comes naturally. Voice your concerns about contaminants in America's food supply to grocers and affect change with dollar power. New York City is legally flushing hydrogenated oils down the garbage disposal, and high fructose corn syrup terrorists are stewing about its future. Corn sugar, *bwa-ha-ha-ha?* A rose by any other name is still dog-doo. Don't be fooled by the corn porn propaganda. You're smarter than that.

If label ingredients read like components of jet fuel, gently drop the container, step away from the shelf and no one will be hurt. Instead, choose the quality building blocks of whole foods for your glorious Holy Temple to achieve health on its own, without chemicals disguised as "natural," wink-wink, food additives.

My grandchildren tell me that if you light a Twinkie on fire, it will burn for 20 minutes. That should "unnaturally" clinch it for you. Getting it?

46
"Natural" My Butt

FDA! You've got PT Barnum twirling in his sarcophagus with glee. Have you been suckered into buying a product declaring itself 100 percent natural? Please! Big Food is acutely aware consumers interpret foods labeled such as wholesome and they exploit it. Kowtowing to lobbyists, the FDA has re-written and holds hostage Webster's dictionary with its contrived, semantic interpretation of "natural". Chew on this: "natural" is not always a synonym for healthful. Under their weak definition, cat poop could be classified as natural.

I just read *"Food Labeling Chaos: The Case for Reform,"* by the Center for Science in the Public Interest (CSPI). The unclear term "natural" sells everything from pet food to ketchup. It's not regulated and probably can't be because by definition, "all natural" can mean almost anything the manufacturer wants it to mean, including nothing at all. The FDA has no plans in the near future to establish a definition of the term "natural" stating, "We have other priorities for our limited resources." Dear readers, don't presume anything and trust no one. Depending on the FDA to protect us is an antiquated notion considering the shocking spate of on-going E. coli and Salmonella outbreaks, carbon monoxide and toxins allowed in our food and pharmaceutical recalls of drugs arrogantly declared harmless. *Sigh...*

The Food Safety and Inspection Service of the USDA requires "natural" to be free of artificial colors, flavors, sweeteners, preservatives and ingredients not occurring naturally in the food. "High fructose corn syrup can't be considered natural and should not be labelled as such," the FDA blurted. So, put down the natural Snapple and no one will get hurt. Archer Daniels Midland Company "convinced" the FDA to reconsider, even though manufacturing HFCS requires a synthetic fixing agent called glutaraldehyde. *"This is very good news, and makes it clear once again that HFCS is at a parity with sugar,"* said the defensive Corn Refiners Association of America. Illiterately irresponsible human behavior, bearing in mind medical literature connects 60 chronic ailments to sugar consumption: cancer, asthma, obesity, allergies, weak immune protection, diabetes and heart disease, hence attractive to the highly profitable medical fraternity. Are they culling the herd of, as BP put it during the Gulf Oil insanity, the small people; the 99 percent?

Non-toxic artificial flavor means anything added for flavor that's not taken directly from whole foods. Ironically, savory, synthetic flavoring chemicals, though unabashedly unnatural, are acceptable in all restrictive diets from vegan to kosher because they're neither animal nor vegetable. Caveat Emptor.

Safe colors exempt from certification include pigments derived from natural sources such as vegetables, or minerals. Examples of exempt colors include annatto extract (yellow), dehydrated beets (bluish-red to brown), real caramel (yellow to tan), beta-carotene (yellow to orange) and grape skin extract (red, green). Consumer activists have said synthetic colors are linked to increased hyperactivity and worsening ADD in innocent children; the secret shame of Big Food and should be banned by FDA. The CSPI and activist groups have formally petitioned the FDA to require a warning label on foods containing any, and appeal for an outright ban on the man-made colors which are toxic to the Holy Temple.

Another widely abused semantic phrase is "made with whole grains." I've encouraged good folks to eat whole grains for 20 years. However, if you use Thomas's Hearty Grains English Muffins or 365 Brand Organic 'Mighty' Multigrain bread, they sound good, however, they contain mostly white flour and a token amount of coarse whole wheat flour, so please reconsider. Read labels. Sandi and I stopped eating wheat gluten and feel so much better. Orchestrated disinformation rules advertising. Look for "Whole Grain" as the first ingredient. Try Ezekiel or Rudi's bread, brown rice, or breads using oats, brown rice, legume flour, or quinoa.

The truth can be illusive and ugly: we're being methodically conned. Virtually anyone can package and market a product to make it sellable, just as you can put lipstick on a pig. But that doesn't show much love for your fellow man.

47
Dietary Self-Destruction?

With the crashing thud of incredulity, my jaw hit the overly polished floor of the Cardio Catheterization lab.

Due to an imperfect artificial heart valve, I occasionally need to be electronically jolted out of atrial fib into normal rhythm; rebooted. This time there was this rotund guy in the next bay being consoled by his wife before his jolt. Whilst receiving his instructions prior to a stent procedure to unblock his clogged arteries, the sweet nurse asked what prescriptions he was taking (12) and what he desired to eat after surgery. He paused, hummed and hawed, then landed on biscuits and gravy, bacon, hash browns and coffee with cream. "What the...?" I stammered under my breath. In 1988 after I kissed the dark scepter of death on the lips and lived to tell of it, I was abundantly motivated to educate myself and then to responsibly change my diet perceptions. But everyone is different; some stronger, some weaker. I joyously share when you change your plate, you change your fate. Then, as if that wasn't sufficient to reboot my heart, I gazed up and witnessed an attractive elderly gal shuffling in for cardiac rehab toting a bag of burgers, fries and a milk shake. Holy crap, they just can't make the profound connection between food and disease. Chew on this: Homicide is 0.8% of deaths. Diet related disease is over 60%, but no one talks about it. Bless their hearts; don't they notice they're eating the same foods that ushered them into poor health? I was stunned but hardly speechless, and if you knew me, you'd appreciate the significance of that statement. In the age of uber-information, it's heartbreaking to watch decent, good-hearted folks continue ladling into the savory stew of ill health and then grumble how much they spend on pharmaceuticals and heart surgery. Not to mention how this all elevates the cost of healthcare for everyone.

According to the CDC, nearly a quarter of all Americans between 20 and 75 percent have hypertension while roughly 70 percent of those over 75 have it. Hypertension is caused by little or no exercise, poor diet, obesity, older age but rarely genetics. Foods which set you up for heart disease are commercial butter from corn-fed bovines, animal renderings, bacon, bologna, hot dogs, gravy, cream sauce, non-dairy creamers, sugar, hydrogenated margarine, shortening, cocoa butter found in chocolate, cottonseed and palm-kernel oils and most ingredients lurking in chain restaurant pantries.

Yes, I'm an unabashed zealot, so when I'm driving down a busy highway and see the endless hodgepodge of chain restaurants brimming with gaggles of rotund folks, or when I enter a Steak and Shake for tea and watch an elderly gal with a tripod walker and oxygen tank struggle to get to a booth, then orders chili fries, I cringe in sad bewilderment. Either they don't read, or they've simply given up because they believe they cannot succeed. One would assume the proposition of death would be ample motivation, but apparently not. Today's food is too addictive. Literally. Science has proven these "bad" foods temporarily make us feel groovy and of course, everyone wants to feel good. The question we must ask ourselves; is a moment of instant gratification worth a $60,000 ICU rendezvous, freaking out your family or worse?

It's up to us to fend off the temptation of harmful foods we've been brainwashed to eat all our lives. We're a malleable bunch.

Disease takes years to manifest itself, so making small changes now can be the best preventive measure. Is it time for you to wean yourself off particular foods scientifically reputed to cause disease and death? Are you motivated into embracing our innate, preordained diet set forth by a generous, loving Creator? It would seem the tasty solution to this challenge is to get out of our own way. Do you get it? I sincerely hope so. I know you can do it! It breaks my heart to see good folks digging their grave with their forks and knives.

48
Taking Risks: The Human Love Affair

Humans have an extraordinary fondness for their small sins and faults. This is why some earthlings refuse, regardless of the truth or outcome, to adapt for their own good.

I once spoke to a seniors group seeking knowledge to improve their health in order to decrease health care expenses. You could've knocked me over with a sugar packet at the rich aroma of palpable denial when I pontificated on the scientific truths that sugar, our beloved American icon, is addictive and poisonous to humans. I squirmed and shuddered as they began lighting torches, gathering feathers, and warming the tar. One woman didn't want to hear the truth about her best friend sugar, copped an attitude and walked out.

Sugar, technically a drug, carries so much socialization and romanticism that good people view it fundamentally different from other kinds of food. Actually, over the past 30 years, America has developed such a great love affair with sugar that it seems natural to include sugar, lots of it, in the diet. Our affaire de Coeur with sugar will go down in history as the greatest mistake of the century. Just like love, caffeine, alcohol, crack, meth, white flour and nicotine, sugar is addictive, and if you don't want to believe me, I double-dog dare you to stop eating it for a week. Sugar has addicted millions of Americans, drawing them into its cruel, debilitating grasp.

It's a non-nutritive, empty calorie that robs the Temple of basic vitamins and minerals needed to sustain health. It has many appellations, such as granulated table sugar, powdered sugar, brown sugar, corn syrup, dextrose, raw sugar, Turbinado, and malt. Refined sugar is a sticky substance, and if left in the bloodstream instead of being burned as energy, sticks to cells. Scientists advise sugar causes premature aging and weakens the Temple's protective immune system, which is not-so-good news during flu and cold season. The white stuff causes obesity, wrinkled skin, dry hair and skin, high triglycerides, high cholesterol, sticky blood platelets, duodenal ulcers, pesky yeast over growth, kidney and liver enlargement, cancer, PMS, cavities, obesity, contributes to diabetes, weakened eyesight, eczema in children, cataracts, emphysema, increased fluid retention, and well, whew, there's simply not enough space here to mention them all. So visit: www.healingcancernaturally.com/sugar-health-effects-risks.

The ugliest part of aging is the appearance of our wrinkling, creeping splotchy skin. Reduce the amount you eat and you'll soon notice a positive change in your hide. The reason is refined carbohydrates such as white bread and other white flour products high in sugar cause delightful skin inflammation. This creates high levels of free radicals which attack the collagen that keeps skin firm. Without sufficient collagen, you'll start to wrinkle.

The diabetes crisis is a result of our country's sugar epidemic, which brings me to share that I dressed up on Halloween as a distressed pancreas. Sorry to say, the average American consumes close to 32 teaspoons of sugar each day or according to the USDA, thirty-one, 5 pound bags annually. Just one can of soda contributes 13 teaspoons, and I ask how often you'd sit down and eat that much intentionally. Sugar is veiled in many foods under the name of high-fructose corn syrup (HFCS), so do your health a favor and be aware of what you put in your indiscriminate, albeit drooling mouth. Cut back or avoid processed sugar and HFCS which are acid-forming and cause problems with digestion, inflammation, gallbladder, as well as reducing your immune systems protective abilities by up to a whopping 92 percent.

By eliminating, sugar, bad fats and empty carbs from your diet, you could almost kiss chronic health diseases good bye. Wouldn't that be a blessing? You might also eliminate costly medications, however, never quit meds without doctor approval. You'll feel better, healthier, plus you'll lose weight. Make a mindful, educated decision today to rid your Holy Temple of the No 1 killer in America, and as I always urge, eat wisely my friends. You are worthy and beautiful.

49
Vegaholics Anonymous

"Hello, my name is Bill and I'm a Vegaholic. *Hi Bill!" "*No matter how hard I try, I can't say no to the rush I get from eating vegetables, any vegetables; my green fix. For gosh sakes, they're virtually everywhere, easy to score at back-alley farmers' markets, salad bars and grocery produce aisles."

His head falls in shame, "Out of sight, behind drawn shades, I greedily eat them with reckless abandon. Life without veggies isn't worth livin'." I'm pathetic, but it makes me feel so darn good-really, really good. You see, I'm addicted to the taste of life. Without vegetables surging through my veins, I will surely wither, withdraw and perish. My baffled family physician mistakenly assumes I'm avoiding him since I never darken his door. I can't help myself; vegetable side-effects arouse my immune system. My meat-munching macho friends call me a weak sissy. But you know what? I couldn't care less. I've never felt groovier." No one forced Bill to become a tree-hugging, grass-eating, granola-crunching vegaholic. It just happened.

Is your Holy Temple whispering to dose-down your red meat intake? Like a hungry python in a bunny cage, are you sucking down processed foods seven days a week from the local convenience store, pushers of low-grade nutrition? That small, tugging voice is your freshly altered mind "Jonesing" for the enjoyable, addictive ecstasy of vegetables. Any veggie junkie will attest there ain't nothin' like the real thing, baby. Our vegaholic friend advises, "Don't buy the bogus GMO vegetables, man. They've like, been stepped-on, man, and don't give you the groovy health buzz. Get an organic connection, dude."

Recently, a gentleman stopped me to say he heeded the plant-based eating advice and capitulated to "vegaholism." He'd lost 30 gut-busting pounds, rarely gets ill, and has refreshed energy-stash and mind-blowing mental clarity. He was a joyfully changed man, a vegetable-dependent junkie glowing with health and self-esteem. Vegaholics live seven years longer than carnivores and have appreciably reduced rates of obesity, coronary heart disease, hypertension, type II diabetes, diet-related cancers, and diverticular disease, constipation, rheumatoid arthritis and gall stones.

Personally I didn't get it. Instead, "it" got me. After surviving terminal heart disease, I began to score more veggies. I began to crave more and more varieties of vegetables, instead of the stepped-on, industrialized, GMO foods which caused me a visit to the "ICU Flop House." Vegetables were merely a bothersome obligatory addendum to a meal. Over time, however, I, too, became a blissed-out veggie junkie.

We are herbivorous. Our composition and digestive system demonstrate that humans have evolved for millions of years living on fruits, nuts, grains, and vegetables. Scientists agree early humans were fruit and vegetable eaters, and throughout history our anatomy has not changed, but our low-grade American diet certainly has turned into tasty nothingness. Man's structure, external and internal, compared with that of the other animals, shows that fruit and succulent vegetables constitute his natural food. As much as some folks detest the addictive "green" stuff, all plant foods have an enormous impact on your Holy Temple. Get-off on these tips:

- Most veggie junkies hook up with a "hoe," and grow their own.
- Farmers markets are veggie junkie "crack houses." You can always count on high-quality stuff.
- Score seasonal fresh fruits. It's cheaper. Plus fresh produce gets you-off better because of their head-spinning nutrition; a natural high.
- Make a plan with your closest enablers and get-off together.

Open your mind, arteries, and mouths to the heavenly buzz of the universal apothecary of plant foods. It's not so much that we are what we eat, but what our Holy Temple absorbs from the pleasurably addictive veggies we were designed to consume by creation.

50
Less is Moo, (Moo or Less)

Since man stood upright then discovered fire, humans have eagerly consumed flame-grilled flesh and will likely continue until the last animal on earth is gone or secreted in fear and dread of man.

Considered socially macho by today's society, the long shadow of uber meat consumption greatly stresses our shared environment. Stewards of earth anxious about climate change already know one of the more significant changes a person can make to their greening lifestyle is reducing excessive meat consumption.

A recent UN report states the typical meat-heavy American diet adds considerably to pollution, water scarcity, land degradation, and climate change. Happily, increased public consciousness of meat-associated health and environmental hazards is having a greening-effect on Americans' dietary behavior. One ginormous source of global warming is the inhumane industrialized factory farming of animals. Because they're a different species than humans is not justification for their slaughter and torment any more than racial, ethnic, or gender differences explain the torment and slaughter of humans. *"Whenever the rainbow appears I will see it and remember the everlasting covenant between God and all living creatures of every kind on the earth."*(Genesis 9:16)

It's undeniable, bovine digestive flatulence contributes to global warming. Methane released from mass-produced bovine gulags contributes a robust portion of greenhouse gases released into our precious atmosphere. While cows in the wild naturally produce methane, they would not exist in such huge, dense populations. Bite by bite America's unquenchable supersized lust for commercial Factory Farmed beef, and lots of it bub, trashes planet earth. Americans dig their graves and plundering earth with knives and forks. (www.factoryfarming.com)

The EPA estimates more than 50 percent of global methane emissions are related to human-related activities. Additionally, it takes about four and a half times the amount of land to grow feed for cattle, versus using the same land to grow local, sustainable sun-blessed plant food ready for consumption. Raising livestock en masse requires more fertilizer and emits more greenhouse gases which have devastating environmental impacts. Local farmers are eternally more environmentally conscious, use less aberrant chemicals, and feed the furry, four-footed ruminants the grass diet set forth by the intelligence of the infinite universe.

Go ahead and have a cow, but before submitting to a daily macho cheese burger, consider the health of our planet as well as its inhabitants. Abstaining eating a cheeseburger today won't reduce global warming tomorrow. Rather, as less meat is consumed, less livestock will be raised, ergo less environmental injury. What's important here is considering what's on your plate each meal and then instituting small, enlightened changes. As a family, consider preparing juicy locally procured grass-fed burgers and stimulate your local economy.

Switching to a more vegetable-based diet will have a delicious impact on our fertile water planet. The number of vegetarians proliferates nationwide, especially among the better-educated and a new generation of young, up-and-coming eco-warriors. The Meatless Monday program is not about turning everyone into vegetarians, but reducing meat consumption by about 15 percent. It's a simple strategy: go meatless for one day every week. The campaign is endorsed by more than 20 schools of public health, including Carnegie Mellon University, Columbia and Harvard; and celebrities like Texan Lance Armstrong, race car driver Leilani Munter and Chef Mario Batali. Presidents Wilson, Truman and Roosevelt galvanized the nation with voluntary meatless days during both world wars, so it's not necessarily a new-fangled concept.

Becoming a flexitarian, vegetarian, vegan or even rawist is one of the single most effective lifestyle changes one can make to mitigate the cancer of global warming. It is unbiased rational thought, curiosity, healthy skepticism and critical inquiry that further a greater harmony and healing. While the prolonged interaction with today's uptight and angry Earthlings may be mind-numbing and fatiguing, the best cure for our ills in life is a walking meditation in loving symbiosis with the sights, sounds, and smells of nature and just let it be.

51
The Haunting Truths about Sugar

When the eerie annual Halloween adulation of the sugar gods draws neigh, please seize a moment to consider what occurs to your ghastly, ghostly bedecked youngster's exquisite inner ecosystem when so much sugar enters his or her young blood stream. It hits their pleasure centers and brain like crack cocaine. This applies to Easter and nearly every American holiday.

There are myriads of truths some good folks would prefer to simply go away, the ignorance-is-bliss approach to life. For the sake of our loved ones, there are however, profundities which shouldn't be sugar-coated. The American Journal of Clinical Nutrition warns sugar stifles the immune system, impairing your defenses against bacteria, virus and infection. Just one teaspoon shuts down the immune system for one hour. Think what happens when you drink a can of cola that contains 13 teaspoons of the nasty, addictive white stuff.

Moms and Dads, researchers at the National Cancer Institute report only one in five precious children consume the recommended minimum of five fruits and vegetables a day, while the top 10 sources of carbohydrates in children's diets include the sugary soft drinks, cakes, cookies, jam and fruit drinks you buy for them. Another study from Tulane University reported children who eat lots of sugar consume significantly lower amounts of protein, vitamins E and D, the B vitamins, iron and zinc.

They also state sugar can cause a rapid rise of adrenaline, hyperactivity, anxiety, difficulty concentrating, and crankiness. The white substance can produce a significant rise in total cholesterol, triglycerides and bad cholesterol and a decrease in good cholesterol. They warn sugar feeds cancer cells and has been connected with the development of cancer of the breast, ovaries, prostate, rectum, pancreas, biliary tract, lung, gallbladder and stomach. Why Big Food hasn't acted more rapidly on this is astonishingly immoral.

"Big Food." as First Lady Michele Obama calls them, has known for decades the ghostly white stuff is addictive, but have profited greatly from the socialized, albeit legal addiction. They even invented lilting mascots to lure you into the alleged Americana culture of comfort-food wholesomeness. Comfort for their bottom line, nevertheless. Once considered irrefutable, the Standard American Diet, covertly contrived by greedy bankers and wealthy commodity brokers, is insidiously based upon the concept of human addiction, not optimum nutrition. You'd be blind not to see the cacophonous maelstrom of beguiling advertising images of coffee, sugar, diet cola, cigarettes, AP flour, booze, saturated animal fats, and yes, milk chocolate.

If you're skeptical, the sweet substance is addictive. In 2002, the American Psychological Society announced, "Evidence exists that even intermittent, excessive sugar intake causes endogenous Opioid Dependence." Opioids are substances that bind to or otherwise affect the opiate receptors on the surface of the human cell. Sugar causes human biochemistry to manufacture the opiate, dopamine, the "feel good" drug. Now you're privy to the truth why you gravitate towards your not-so best friend, sugar, when you're singing the blues and feeling scrawny. It makes you high, gets you off, and then you naturally crave more...now! Just like street drugs. Zoom, crash, and burn.

Recently the American Heart Associate announced Americans are consuming too much sugar. Just pay attention to the daily CNN and local news reports. One-half the total weight of a box of Raisin Bran for example, is sugar. The American Diabetes Association says many children get an average of 20 percent of their daily calories from sugar. That means children average 29 teaspoons (one ounce) of added refined sugar per day under non-Halloween conditions. Plus, every year, teens eat an average of 93 pounds of added refined sugar. It's anyone's guess how much they eat on Halloween and the pancreas-stressing days ahead. This year I'm dressing up as a distressed Pancreas to collect money for the ADA and handing out insulin.

52
Here Comes "D" Sun Food

Our 4.5 billion-year-old sun, the axis of the universe, fathers all life. Sunbeams provide nutrition for vegetation eaten by omnivores then consumed by other animals, ultimately consumed by humans and so on and so forth. Since the creation of Earth, the cycle of all life has obtained power and energy from the sun. Without sol's warm rays, Earth could not support life.

Sunlight is considered the best source for vitamin D. When aging kicks in, we spend more time indoors. Outdoors we slather on sun screen, blocking wavelengths that stimulate the Holy Temple to synthesize vitamin D. Subsequently, the *Archives of Internal Medicine* report 77 percent of Americans are vitamin D-ficient linked to high blood pressure, depression, weak immune system, diabetes, poor lung function, autism, fibromyalgia, schizophrenia, MS, osteoarthritis and RA. Not a sunny picture. The major biological function of D is to maintain normal blood levels of calcium and phosphorus. It also supports all organs plus 2,000 genes and in concert with a number of other vitamins, minerals and hormones, promote bone mineralization. Without D, bones become thin, brittle, soft or misshapen. Those who stopped taking statins because of leg pain, The New England Journal of Medicine implicate D-ficiency as the cause. Vitamin D diminishes risk of cancers, autoimmune diseases, infectious diseases, cardiovascular disease and early age-related macular degeneration, especially D-3.

If you're an easy mark for flu, colds, sinus and bronchial infections, or pneumonia, vitamin D-3 regulates T-cells and is absolutely indispensable for a protective immune system. Put this in context with winter colds, sniffles, flu and depression and ...sigh... it's all too clear why we're a sickly bunch. My dear family, including my 93-year-old mom told me she took 5000 IU D-3 daily over the last two winters and never had so much as a sniffle.

The RDA for D established 60 years ago is an insignificant 400 IU when it should've been 10 times higher. But our leaders failed miserably researching basic human nutrition standards. They were satisfied there was a Pharma pill for every ill. RDA stands for Recommended Dietary Allowances, a "norm" established by the FDA during World War II. It was intended to provide educated guidelines for how much of particular nutrients a normal, healthy person requires to stay fit and healthy. The Canadian Cancer Society responsibly upped its advice to 1,000 IU's a day. Others believe northern climates should consume at least 2,000 IU's a day. "The first thing we'd see is a reduction by 80 percent in the incidence of type 1 diabetes," said Cedric Garland, a professor of family and preventive medicine at the University of California at San Diego. "The next thing we'd see is a reduction by about 75 percent of all invasive cancers combined, as well as similar reductions in colon cancer and breast cancer, and probably about a 25 percent reduction in ovarian cancer."

Salmon, tuna, mackerel and fish liver oils are among the best dietary sources of D. Cows moo loudly that their milk's fortified with D but it's synthetic rubbish. Minute amounts of D exists in grass-fed beef liver, cheese and organic, free-range egg yolks. Vitamin D in these foods is primarily in the form of vitamin D_3.

During the warm parts of the year our magnificent Holy Temple produces the "sunshine" vitamin from 10 minutes of daily rays, but ol' sol dips lower on the fall and winter horizon not returning till late spring to bathe the Earth's needy Northern hemisphere. Northern United States is so dark in winter, D synthesis shuts down completely. If for some reason you're unable to eat foods with D or to get enough sunlight, Dr. Chuck Landon, PhD, ND, DaHOM of Indianapolis suggests taking 2,000 to 10,000 IU daily. No adverse effects have been seen with supplemental vitamin D-3 intakes up to 50,000 IU daily. Skip the counterfeit, synthesized grocery crap from China and support your community vitamin store. For most Caucasians, a half-hour in the summer sun in a bathing suit can initiate the release of 50,000 IU vitamin D into the circulation within 24 hours of exposure. This same amount of exposure yields 20,000–30,000 IU in tanned individuals and 8,000–10,000 IU in dark-skinned people. While the study focused on white Americans, the same geographical trend affects black Americans whose overall cancer rates are significantly higher. Darker skinned people require more sunlight to synthesize the vitamin.

Americans have been hard-wired to blindly believe more is better of anything, hence the skin cancer paradox. While it's true the sun isn't a wonder drug, it's elemental in sustaining human health. The benevolent giver has been worshipped by many cultures throughout history because of its vast healing and therapeutic powers. At the turn of the century, people considered the sun good for health and touted it as a cure for major disease. It was a time when "recuperating in the sun" grew popular, claiming extensive exposure, preferably by the seaside, was a magical cure-all for plague, old age and TB.

It's so very correct there's nothing new under the sun. So, get 10 minutes of sun, than apply the gooey white stuff and go out and let the sunshine bathe your beautiful skin. After sun sets, coat your exposed skin with soothing, healing virgin, unrefined coconut oil.

53
Change: A Necessary Evil

"How dare you propose I stop eating the way my parents taught me? If it was good enough for them, by-golly, it's good enough for me." As the kids today articulate, that's lame.

Accepting earthlings' imperfect humanness, everyone struggles letting go of comforting family rituals: stepping outside their dietary comfort zone. At the grocery, folks instinctively reach for expedient sources of food. Ergo, for their daily 3-squares, Americans suckle on the teats of Big Food's rubbish, not honest home cookin' made with love. As a result we've become a sickly bunch due to the proliferation of abnormal man-made substances our cells can't utilize to sustain a healthy Holy Temple. The more fresh food gets altered, the sicker a nation becomes. If we are not healthy, we're not happy. If we're not healthy, we're powerless to contribute to the betterment of society. When we're not healthy, we exhibit disrespect for the Holy Temple, the home of our wandering soul.

Isaac Asimov was quoted, "The only constant is change, continuing change, inevitable change that is the dominant factor in society today. No sensible decision can be made any longer without taking into account not only the world as it is, but the world as it will be."

We like things just the way they are, thank you. Strangely enough, we vainly modify our fashion styles, hair and make-up, and our cars, but give precious little thought to modifying the un-holy dietary assault on the Holy Temple with dead, albeit convenient food. "I've lived this long, why should I change now?" At 90, small dietary changes open up a big ol' can of "feel good." Living is breathtakingly sacred; why would anyone, for the sake of flavor, compromise life's worth.

Before the Industrial Revolution, American communities bartered, shared, canned fresh food, and constructed supportive, peaceful communities centered on local family farms bursting with sustainable sun-blessed produce. Dairy farmers and bee keepers, fed their celestially buddies their divine diet. One-hundred years ago everyone knew local farmers by their first name, shaking their calloused milking hand as they greeted. An ecologically centered community knits itself together with threads of peace and friendship through the sharing of home-made foods simmered with loving energy.

Grandma would have a conniption if she knew folks today eat laboratory-altered food fare shipped from a factory 2,000 miles away. Next time you grocery shop, inspect the shelves creaking from the burden of faux foods and then ask yourself, "Did these foods exist 100 years ago?" If you took every food off the grocer's shelves that didn't exist back then, they'd be bare.

Big Food con artists thrill suckering you into buying their products so they use bright colors on the packages and inviting photos of the products, and they may make some sort of barely supportable health claim on the label. Yes, they're appealingly merchandised, but are you really looking at them for what they truly are, or have you become emotionally and robotically habituated to Betty Crocker and Uncle Ben? We become comfortably numb with the grocery milieu and don't take kindly to change; it freaks folks out, forcing them to examine the purity and source of food and its overall effects on the Holy Temple.

We've witnessed mind-blowing changes in our eating habits during our numerous trips around the sun, and I'm beginning to believe many of these changes are causing the wheels to come off our cherished American way of life. Nothing has changed more than America's farming procedures, food production methods, and the grocery store experience. Even though we know a certain food damages our Temple, curiously, it seems to be the new norm where folks exhibit no compunction, consuming insalubrious, pre-made foods constructed by a cold, steely machine. You know better.

Remember the joyous act of cooking from scratch? Familiarity may or may not breed contempt, but it undeniably breeds comfort. Change doesn't have to be bad. Change for the better is good. Change in the way we eat causes delicious changes in others. Be the solution. To eat is a necessity, but to eat intelligently is an art.

54
Breakfast with 'Cereal' Killers

The road to perdition is paved with good intentions. Did you know Kellogg invented breakfast cereal by accident? Chew on this: the brothers were actually trying to create a bread replacement for inmates at the Battle Creek (Michigan) Sanatorium. Created as a "health food," the Kellogg brothers added sugar to the mix, then marketing executives got busy and the rest is history.

According to author and food historian Andrew F. Smith in AlterNet.org, "Cold cereals are an invention of vegetarians and the health-food industry, first through Kellogg's and then through C.W. Post, which steals all of Kellogg's ideas. These companies realized early on that people like sugar, and kids really like sugar, so they shifted their sales target from adults concerned about health to kids who love sugar. It's an American invention." Are humans predatory by nature?

Today's cereals are senselessly high in toxic sugar composed of processed, sweetened GMO grains peppered with useless synthetic vitamins. Volumes of peer-reviewed studies support the disparaging effects of sugar on the sacred Holy Temple. Even "healthy" low-sugar cereals are dietary boondoggles; both spike blood sugar and insulin.

The Weston Price Foundation says, "Dry breakfast cereals are produced by a process called *extrusion*. Cereal makers first create a slurry of grains and then put them in an *extruder*. The grains are forced out of a little hole at high temperature and pressure. Depending on the shape of the hole, the grains are made into little o's, flakes, animal shapes, or shreds (as in Shredded Wheat or Triscuits), or they are puffed (as in puffed rice). A blade slices off each little flake or shape, which is then carried past a nozzle and sprayed with a coating of oil and sugar to seal off the cereal from the ravages of milk and to give it crunch."

I suggest Ezekiel bread spread with organic tahini, almond or peanut butter. How about plain organic coconut yogurt with real fruit, ground flax or chia seed and nuts, or local eggs with avocado and salsa, vegetable juice, or a fruit and vegetable blender smoothie? Just say "no" to Tony the Tiger.

55
Aging with Grace and Style

Last weekend, seduced by earth's autumn splendor, azure skies, and crisp air, Sandi and I traveled rolling, country back roads through Bear Wallow to visit granddaughter Brittany as she attends her third year at Indiana University. In the midst of all that youth, despite my steadfast aerobic work-out routine and diet, I truly felt the droopy 67- year-old man I accept and love. I mean, wasn't it last year I cradled her in my arms as she cooed and giggled, yanked off my glasses while dutifully filling her diapers?

Life is a terminal disease. Face it, we're all going to die, although decisions you make between birth and death factor grandly into the outcome of life's final scenes. Am I going to experience late-life morbidity or wake up dead some morning? Using this stimulus, appraise your efforts to steward the Holy Temple to stay healthy until you expire. Living to 100 is not attractive unless you make an effort to remain in lucid mental and physical health and keep learning.

After overcoming cancerous cigarette addiction, my first focus was losing weight and keeping it off; the most important thing anyone can do to live longer. Fat cells produce hormones which raise the risk of type 2 diabetes and generate inflammation, stiffening of the arteries, heart, some cancers, and other organs.

Take multivitamins? Big Pharma would love the vitamin industry to go away, thank you. Out of fear and greed, for decades they've unjustly slandered and diminished vitamin and mineral supplement efficacy. Yes, there are substandard vitamins out there, but after some homework and friending a clerk at your community vitamin shop, anyone can deduce good from bad. Grocery store and pharmacy vitamins are the worst. Most are synthesized by Big Pharma or a Chinese chemist, not sourced from our Creator.

The University of California Berkley reports golden agers should take a daily, food-based multiple vitamin with minerals. Women over 50 should take 1,500 mg calcium / magnesium / potassium blend daily and men over 50, 800. They recommend taking daily doses of 800 mg alpha-lipoic acid and 2,000 mg acetyl-l-Carnitine, nutritional warriors that power aging cells. Mitochondrion decay is a major factor in aging and is connected to Alzheimer's and diabetes. Anyone over 50 should also pop a B-Complex and 10,000 IU's D-3 every other day.

You can chill without a pill. Rediscover the ancient practice of taking in and releasing a series of deep, cleansing breaths. Life's stressors increase the concentration of hormones cortisol and norepinephrine which raises blood pressure and suppress immune function. Turn off the TV and computer then seek daily quiet time to meditate and breathe. Begin by centering on each breath. Exhale strongly, making a throaty whoosh sound. Breathe in quietly through the nose for a four count. Hold the breath for a one count, and then exhale with the whoosh sound for a six count. Repeat the cycle four more times and feel the increased oxygen refresh mind, body and soul. Dr. Andrew Weil says deep breathing is a universal anti-stress practice.

Do you still throw a hissy-fit and refuse to eat your fruits and vegetables? Put your big boy pants on vegaphobes; respect your Holy Temple! You're rusting, my wrinkling, and oxidizing friends. Antioxidants in fresh, sun-blessed produce are indispensable as we age as they give the bum's rush to inflammation and free radicals oxidation (rust) that damages healthy cells. This includes all green leafy fibrous and vigorous vegetables such as lettuce, spinach, collards and kale, carrots, sprouts, cucumbers, sweet potatoes, avocado, and celery.

It's wondrous how our Holy Temple intelligence heals and restores. The best kept secret in mainstream medicine is that under the right conditions, your Temple can heal itself.

People live longer today than ever, partly due to savings-sucking life-support machines and what scientists and doctors are discovering Holy Temple chemistry responds to a diet rich in anti-aging garden produce, eager to prolong your relatively short Earth life. As a final point: perform unselfish deeds daily. The best way to stay in a calm, mentally healthy state of bliss is to be kind, accepting, compassionate and loving to others, and to your Holy Temple. And breathe deeply.

56
Macho Doesn't Mean Mucho: Man up!

Shopping recently, I came upon a stressed and bewildered gal examining the shelves of the grocery healthy foods section as if was another galaxy. Looking at me with pleading eyes, she solicited, "Do you know anything about these foods?" Like a famished cat offered a bowl of milk, she eagerly accepted my help.

"Well, my fat, stubborn, macho, diabetic husband refuses to eat anything but potatoes, red meats, butter, bacon, beer, sugar, and white bread," she carped, "He thinks corn and green beans are the only vegetables on earth. His doctor warned if he doesn't alter his meat and potato diet, he'll stroke out precipitating an early rendezvous with his Maker! I'm genuinely frightened."

As a motivational speaker, nutritional literacy educator and researcher, I hear this lament far and wide. Macho Men are resistant to change within their stereotypical masculine diet. Consequentially, loving wives live uneasily with the grim prospect of losing partners and providers. Over the decades, most men have been brainwashed that meat three times a day is macho and vegetables are for sissy boys.

For 16 years our catering firm fed the Pacers charter aircraft and every NBA team they played. I remember early on when he was an immature, cocky rookie, Reggie Miller entering the chartered 727 with a box of Milky Way's, Ding Dong's, and a quart of Mountain Dew, aka, Country Cousin Champagne. Slumped, metabolizing, and sweaty, the players ridiculed our buffet of fresh veggies, real sliced turkey breast, humus, guacamole, and boiled shrimp. Rik Smits entered the plane after four grueling quarters defending the hoop, then, to restore his energy, would pick up and suck down at once five baby quiche. I say it takes a macho man to eat vegetables. "Hey, don't kill the caterer!"

Sixteen years later these same thoroughbreds were demanding fresh vegetables, fruits, lean cuts of poultry, beef tenderloin, pork loin instead of chops, grilled salmon fillets without heavy cream sauce, and gave up ordering fried foods. They put on their big-boy pants, became real men, and transcended crappy food, recognizing the more real foods and less artery-lining gelatinous goo they ate, their mental as well as physical, on-court performance, plus their impending trade value dramatically improved. By the 2000 playoffs with the Los Angeles Lakers, there were three savvy Pacers who had become vegetarian. The Lakers had nine. These enlightened "macho" players learned that next to breathing and sleeping, eating is the most important thing you do to sustain your Holy Temple. They opened their minds and realized everything about their entire being was the result of their daily food choices.

Without learning to intelligently select more real foods, they may have never reached mental or physical perfection as the Cosmos generously planned.

In addition, eating more plant foods normalizes blood pressure and promotes cardiovascular health. A recent group study of men with high cholesterol, published in the *Annals of Internal Medicine*, reported a diet high in vegetables, fruits, nuts, and whole grains improved blood flow and prevented damage to cells lining the arteries. Vegetables also improve blood flow, the top secret ingredient of a happy love life since a healthy vascular system is required to prevent the heartbreak of erectile dysfunction, or assault with a dead weapon.

After my grocery buddy and I talked a bit you could see the lights go on and the stress drain from her pretty face. To my thinking, it takes a real man to embrace plant foods and a plant-based diet rather than continuing to suck down self-destructive foods. I totally agree with Zsa Zsa Garbor, "Macho doesn't prove mucho."

57
The Holiday Paradox: Is Gluttony a Sin?

Christmas season kindles treasured childhood reminiscence. Oozy feelings of undiluted love as I snuggled on the couch, enveloped in Mom's heirloom afghan, bathed in the amber-red glow of crackling timber, captivated by surreal, multi-hued petite lights, silvery tensile, and the scent of pine commingling with the aroma of freshly baked holiday goodies. My body tingled in anticipation of the arrival of jolly friends and family strung together like treasured holiday ornaments, decking the house with delicious affection and joy, everyone eager for the Grandma's prayer kicking off the abundant holiday dinner.

These visions conjure humorous post-dinner negotiation for the Barcalounger, menfolk napping, snoring with one eye open while watching the Detroit Lions, and the womenfolk "wired" on caffeine and sugar, speed-talking as their tongues smoldered and swelled. Finally, there was the belt loosening competition, and subsequent bathroom marathon. "Hey, whatcha' readin' in there, *War and Peace*?"

With each family's arrival, the 16 foot buffet table filled with time-honored foods like mashed potatoes oozing with heavy cream and butter, baked ham, roasted chicken, barn animal gravy, deviled eggs, sweet 'taters feloniously assaulted with sugar and marshmallows, broccoli casserole with dried onion rings, green beans simmered 12 hours in pork knuckles, psychedelic gelatin salads, yeast rolls with butter, cheese balls, pecan pies, cookies, candies, and, well the list is infinite. However, fresh vegetables were uninvited. Reflecting, I can't recall anything resembling true nourishment. Actually everything was deliciously unhealthful. However we've become numbly oblivious these foods, in the end trash our Holy Temple, Jesus' abode. Happy Birthday!

I'm not trying to plop reindeer droppings into your eggnog, however, knowing your Holy Temple is God's earthly dwelling place, do you maintain an irreverent, lackadaisical, "I am too busy to consider cooking healthier attitude?" Or, are you a reverential steward of your Holy Temple? Research reveals holiday food traditions damage the Holy Temple, but we've blurred the notion food has anything to do with poor health and that disease is just a natural part of aging; God's will. At 40, we're considered old and ripe for late life disease. Really? It's God's will that we get ill? Not my God.

Food has everything to do with personal stewardship, spiritual connectivity, and mental acuity. While celebrating Christ's birth, our
culture considers over-eating normal. Christians nowadays have forgotten they were charged at birth with the responsibility of personal stewardship, God's greatest creation. I refer to Corinthians 3:16 & 17. *"Do you not understand that you are God's Temple, and that God's Spirit has His permanent dwelling in you? If anyone destroys God's Temple, God will destroy him. For the Temple of God is holy and sacred to Him; and so you, as His Temple are also holy."* Verily I sayeth that's "severeth," but it's in the Good Book. Just like coveting and gluttony, man's selectively edited heavenly commands.

Behold, I bring you tidings of great joy! By replacing head hunger with the will of creation, "Yule" transfer the urge for foods that cause heart disease, diabetes, obesity, and cancer for hungering and thirsting for righteousness and nutritional literacy. The message of faith, love, kindness and compassion will challenge us in our strength and comfort us in our human weakness for un-holy food.

Want to know what I want for Christmas? For everyone to keep their money, pay their bills, and sit down together to enjoy a modest, wholesome, home-cooked meal and enjoy being part of a family. I want to see people refuse to be manipulated by emotionally tinged commercials and two hour-only sales. I want people to put aside greed and status-seeking, and the love of all things material. Instead, I wish everyone would give each other warm, 20-second hugs and be thankful for what they have. I'm confident personal stewardship would be the perfect birthday gift to you.

58
Who Put the Squeeze on OJ?

Orange juice holds position in the hallowed American pantheon of traditional breakfast foods. Each year 620 million gallons of orange ambrosial cure-all are consumed in the U.S. But, is it truly fresh or are you being flim-flamed—again?

Ads pitching today's version of the pulpy juice tell us, *wink, wink,* it's pure and natural so we blindly buy the citrus au jus for the sentiment. Nevertheless, the majority of your American tradition comes, tell-me-it-ain't-so, from sunny Brazil and volatile Mexico. That's emphatically un-Patriotic.

As an OJ drinker you've been misinformed about what you're actually drinking. Most folks get "juiced" when they learn big brands marketing their product as "pure and simple" add flavor packs to revitalize it and make it fresh, once again. "From concentrate" and most "not from concentrate" orange juice undergo processes that strip flavor and nutrition. The largest producers of "not from concentrate" or pasteurized orange juice keep juice in million-gallon aseptic storage tanks to ensure a year round supply. Aseptic storage strips the ethereal juice of oxygen, a process known as deaeration, so the juice doesn't oxidize in the "tank farms" where aging juice sits for as long as a year.

Dubious flavor packs are fabricated from the chemicals that make up orange essence and oil. Flavor and fragrance houses, the same ones making high-end perfume, break down orange essence oils into their constituent chemicals then reassemble the individual chemicals in configurations resembling nothing in nature.

Delicious ethyl butyrate is one of the charming chemicals found in high concentrations in flavor packs. Flavor engineers discovered it imparts a fragrance Americans dig and associate with a fresh squeezed. It's an amoral con job, the American business model.

Wrong on so many levels, Tropicana reformulated its healthy heart juice, adding fish oil, sardines, tilapia, and fish gelatin for the Omega 3 . This makes as much sense as lighting yourself on fire then running naked through a meth lab. Eating fatty fish, ground flax and chia seeds and walnuts is infinitely better.

Orange juice is celebrated as a healthy drink but few realized it contains the same amount of toxic sugar as cola. In the world orange juice market, the leading brand is Tropicana, owned by PepsiCo since 1998. In April 2008 the Journal Diabetes Care studied diets of 70,000 women as part of the Nurse's Health Study. They found that unlike daily consumption of fresh fruit and vegetables associated with an 18 per cent reduction in the risk of diabetes, consumption of fruit juice, even in small daily amounts, was associated with an overall 18 per cent *increased* risk for diabetes. Why are diabetics told they can have just a little sugar? It's like offering a recovering meth addict "just a little." That's insane considering rates of diabetes continue to soar unchecked. It's time medical cowards grow a set and stop pandering for funds and seek a new protocol. Diabetes makes a lot of corporations, executives and drug company's bushels of dirty money.

Vitamin C and its potent cancer protection is the most easily destroyed vitamin there is. It is destroyed by exposure to oxygen and heat (above 70 degrees) Processed, pasteurized OJ (145 °) is a pitiable surrogate for fresh, sun-blessed orange juice squeezed at home from cooperative oranges. Pasteurization obliterates most of the juices' health-sustaining phytonutrients, including anti-cancer nutrients. Heat alters the molecular structure of OJ, creating higher acidity during digestion. Acidity sets us up for cancer and inflammation. And, that's not to mention the enormous natural resources used to process, concentrate, transport, and reconstitute.

If you're the sissy who protests pithy parts, for the love of God and your caring family, get over it. You're a responsible adult now, in charge of your health destiny. That's where all the nutritional goodness lurks, so "orange up." Fresh-squeezed OJ tastes ethereal, and supermarkets do sell it. They charge too much, however. Return to a pre-industrial revolution mentality. Make family time to juice your own. It's vastly cheaper, and your Temple will definitely groove from the purity, hearty nutrition, and wholeness.

No bottle of self-respecting vodka would even want to cozy up to this abomination of the Great Creators unselfish gifts to US. If you can't gather the gumption to squeeze the orange, frozen unsweetened OJ concentrate contains a lot of vitamin C and was not heated. If half the world can, then why can't we? We're lazy and worship convenience, and for that, there's an unpleasant tradeoff.

Big Food and scientist pretending to be chefs will never be able to graft the hand of God. Karma baby, karma.

59
Feed Your Heart's Needs II

When I weighed 300 pounds, an elective lobotomy seemed considerably more tempting than abandoning my beloved American food fare. It was walk away, or meet thy Maker. My uneducated, meat-heavy, deep fried Midwestern mentality came home to roost in the lining of my gelatinous, unexercised heart. A thankful beneficiary of a miracle, I sympathize how easier-said-than-done it is to wave farewell to familiar foods that, over time, destabilize our Temples, causing plaque to narrow and harden arteries. My unbridled lust for refined carbs, gravy, and saturated fat created conditions ripe for a prefect myocardial infarction storm. Thud! 911!

At first it was a series of lasts: the last burger, deep-fried food, jelly doughnut, eggs cooked in bacon grease, sausage gravy, bucket o' chicken parts, and "Poop Tarts." I was bewildered by how many of my enabler-soon-to-be-ex-friends attempted sucking me back into their comfy black vortex of ignorant dietary behaviors that landed me in ICU. "Don't be a sissy, eat some bacon!"

Breaking the chains lashing me to the flagpole of self-destruction was the mightiest life battle I've waged. The near-death experience taught me the proposition of death can be motivating and that our Creator helps those who help themselves. Healthy and whole again, I committed to and embarked upon a life journey of food literacy, which has successfully extended my life and shown a floodlight on my calling.

Other than sloth, the food we eat is a major factor in acquiring or avoiding heart disease. The American Journal of Clinical Nutrition says chronic health problems either wholly or partially credited to a poor diet represent a serious threat to public health. Daily unwholesome eating and inactivity are responsible for more deaths than booze, illicit use of street drugs, sexual behavior, arguing with neighbors over politics, and firearms. Perishing due to an inadequate diet in a land of plenty is unheard of in history! People classically kicked the bucket because of plagues, famines, and wars, not a poor and imbalanced diet.

The Heart and Stroke Foundation taught fresh, local fruits and vegetables reduce inflammation, hardening of the arteries, and lower bad cholesterol. I discovered triglycerides naturally produced by the liver also come from food. The Temple produces excessive triglycerides when ingesting too many refined carbohydrate rich foods containing heart damaging fats and useless calories. Excessive alcohol, smoking and lack of exercise increase triglycerides. Fresh caught, salmon and trout brim with Omega-3 that reduces triglycerides. The groovy oils in these fish increase the good cholesterol. Eat more fibrous foods since they are high-quality sources of heart-healthy antioxidants as well as cholesterol-lowering dietary fiber. Maintain a happy colon to achieve optimum health.

Peanuts, walnuts, and almonds are a healthy snacks packed with protein, vitamins and minerals indispensable to a joyful heart. Raw cacao, not cocoa powder, contains blissful antioxidants that lower blood pressure. Avocado, my favorite, provides fiber, monounsaturated fats, and oleic acid that helps reduce blood pressure spikes triggered by sodium.

After recognizing then conquering each destructive craving, I became stronger, and my self-esteem soared into the heavens. After gaining control of my eating, I'd treat myself to a weekly naughty bit as a reward, not a daily ritual. There was no way I was heading down that road again. No way! Gradually I gained further strength and decided Nietzsche was right; the more you sacrifice and conquer that which destroys you, the stronger and more honest you become with yourselves in all aspects of life.

There are constellations of real, living, highly vibrational foods that prevent and resolve heart disease problems, but purchasing heart healthy food isn't easy these days. Shopping with my grandson recently, he made an astute observation: "If this is the healthy section, grandpa, does that mean the rest of the store is unhealthy stuff?" From the mouths of babes.

Most assume the chambered heart merely pumps blood. Falling in love or grieving is all in the head. Pump, pump. That's all. Au contraire, Mon Fraire, it's our "second brain." One cannot live nor love without it; intimacy and laughter are good for it; bad news can break it; and poor nutrition will trash it.

For centuries, the Valentine-shaped organ's been connected to emotion. Poets and scholars through history were right: the heart houses mind and soul. The Chinese associated hearts with the epicenter of happiness, the Greeks the seat of their spirit. Early Egyptians understood the connection of the heart to the pulse saying it "speaks in the vessels of all the members."

Since both Satan and Jesus knock at its door, the human heart apparently merits tender loving care in many of ways. How do you treat your heart and soul? The 10-ounce heart beats without stopping 24/7/365, decade after decade, therefore when dietary and spiritual needs go unmet, we feel empty, desperate and woozy from a lack of love, proper, natural nourishment and oxygen. The brain needs oxygen and glucose, which, if not received continuously, causes you to lose consciousness. Muscles need glucose, amino acids, sodium, calcium, vitamins, and potassium salts from clean foods to work normally.

A muscle beating roughly 72 times per minute, the heart altruistically pumps life-blood throughout your universe within, shuttling vital materials which sustain mental and physical functions while removing waste products from your ecology. That's why it needs strengthening exercise like all muscles. Like a starving man seeks food, the soul seeks symbiotic satisfaction; you keep me happy and I'll keep you happy. Regardless of creed, we have commonality: hungry hearts. We know the importance of feeding the soul with worship and meditation, but what's it require to operate perfectly as creation intended? Real foods like almonds, apples, beans, blueberry's, avocado, and fresh fish are awesome additions to your daily fare. Food is one of the greatest issues in today's culture; questions about the supply of nourishment for the human race saturate the media. We get so preoccupied with the temporary, we neglect the eternal.

The heart, the core of your existence, makes you tick. It houses your health, Creator, love, joy, and bliss. It's a source of one's being, emotions, and sensibilities as in "an appeal from the heart," or "a man after my own heart." It's the innermost physical core, "It touched my heart," and "in your heat you know it's true." You can also break or touch someone's heart with words or actions. You share sincere heart to hearts, and spiritually feed your heart with the Word, then after church, undo it all by eating fried chicken cooked in pork fat and gravy medical science says block blood flow causing "the big one." Due to this eating tradition, Midwesterners trend above the national average for heart disease and a diseased heart struggles to express the splendor of love.

Laugh at your self-absorbed nature when things get harsh and sidestep grumpy, life-sucking people; social vampires. A hardy laugh warms the soul and increases blood flow for up to 45 minutes after a belly laugh.

Those who have awakened and are paying attention to what they eat are aware what they do or do not put into their Holy

Temple impacts their spiritual well-being and increases connection to our higher cosmic source. The idea is not new. Eastern philosophers and Christian saints have long suggested fasting as penance or to cleanse their bodies, regarded as the Temple of their spirit. Many of Earth's religions have ancient laws forbidding certain foods or combinations of foods as unholy or unclean, contaminating to the Holy Spirit. Unclean = junk food.

Fall in love with yourself with all your heart. Your Holy Temple requires devotion, respect, and educated stewardship for the beat to go on and for Mother Earth to endure man's ignorant parasitical pillage of her diminishing resources.

60
Celery: Ancient, Crunchy Medicine

Let's hear it for Celeryville, Ohio, a hard-working community reputed for their robust, annual celery harvest. Migrating celery farmers first settled there and began cultivating the noble vegetable which has evolved into an indispensable member of America's crisper drawer.

Ancient literature documents celery, a member of the carrots, parsley, dill, fennel, Hemlock and cilantro family, originated in the Mediterranean basin and was cultivated for medicinal purposes before 850 BC. Celery oil was used to treat colds, flu, water retention, and inefficient digestion, various types of inflammatory arthritis, liver and spleen ailments. Ancient Greeks considered celery a holy plant and decorated winners at the Olympic Games using its flavorful leaves as laurels.

Other than a predictable portion of a vegetable tray or a greasy buffalo wings garnish, raw celery is laden with cancer-fighting vitamin C, which fortifies your Holy Temple's immune system, stops cancerous free-radical oxidation, halts the inflammation cascade, and helps reduce cold symptoms or severity of cold symptoms. Over 20 scientific studies have concluded that vitamin C is a cold-fighter. Vitamin C promotes cardiovascular health and can help lower cholesterol levels. Researchers show C's from vegetables and fruits high in this nutrient are associated with a reduced risk of death from all causes including heart disease, stroke and cancer. In some areas celery and celery seed is consumed to treat high blood pressure.

Crispy celery is a very good source of dietary fiber, potassium, folate, molybdenum, manganese and vitamin B6. Celery is also a healthy source of calcium, vitamin B1, vitamin B2, magnesium, vitamin A, phosphorus and iron. Celery also possesses cholesterol lowering benefits. Celery only contains approximately 35 milligrams of sodium per stalk, so salt-sensitive individuals can enjoy celery, but should keep track of this amount when monitoring daily sodium intake. A recent edition of Details magazine reports: "Celery is suspected to be somewhat sexually arousing." and speculates the cause is that: "Celery contains androsterone and pheromone, powerful hormones researchers believe is released through sweat glands and attracts females." Oo-la-la!

It warms my heart chakra to hear of nutritionally food literate mothers who use carrot and celery sticks while their babies teethe, introducing them early in life to nature's sun blest Apothecary. After you "stalk" some down, wash, and wash as if your life depended on it. Conventional and organic celery is grown close to the ground which offers them up for snarky bacterial contamination and animal droppings. Of course, you already knew.

As an all-around maintainer of your Holy Temple's health, celery gets top billing. Celeriac is becoming popular as a part of trendy American gourmet eating. Americans prefer green stalk celery and mainly eat it raw. What's life without occasionally making ants on a log with the grandkids, so crunch away!

61
Too Much Wheat's not so Neat

We associate wheat with apple pie, the American flag, and "God Bless America." Although today the future of wheat is uncertain. Why is there such a strong emphasis on eating wheat products when there are so many adverse and crippling effects such as neurological impairment, dementia, heart disease, cataracts, diabetes, arthritis and visceral fat accumulation, not to mention the full range of intolerances and bloating now experienced by millions of people?

The food pyramid even encourages eating a whopping six to eleven servings a day. Might it be because Grain Foods Foundation lobbyist board members have ties to diabetes and drug manufacturers? Bingo! You can't make this up folks, we eat too much "carbolicious" wheat and it's taking a tragic toll.

Great news! We're witness to a welcome dietary awakening. Medical science is making Americans aware of their self-destructive, blind devotion to unhealthy eating customs, vegaphobia, and dependence on carbs that initiate disease and diminishes their earthly quality of life. Betty Crocker and Tony the Tiger have trained Americans to perceive white flour as healthy, but half the unsaturated fatty acids, EFS's, all the vitamins, fifty percent of the calcium, 70 percent of the phosphorus, 80 percent of the iron, 98 percent of the magnesium, and 50 to 80 percent of the B vitamins are destroyed via industrial strength processing. American's best buddy is linked to diabetes, Celiac Disease, inflammation, accelerated aging, cancer, depression, anxiety, and "poochy" belly.

Wheat's not neat since today it's drastically altered from our Creator's original design and contains a powerful little chemical in known as "wheat germ agglutinin" (WGA), which is largely responsible for many of wheat's pervasive, and difficult-to-diagnose ill effects.

Our Holy Temple struggles with digesting alien strains of wheat and disease happens. According to Dr. David Kessler, retired FDA head asserts modern processed wheat; vastly different from the original earliest forms is addictive, much like crack cocaine, sugar, cigarettes, caffeine and alcohol.

Alloxan, what makes AP flour clean and white, creates free radicals in pancreatic beta cells, thus destroying them and you get diabetes. BTW: Alloxan is given to lab rats to damage the pancreas for studying its toxic effect. Alloxan's effects on the pancreas are so severe the *Textbook of Natural Medicine* calls it "a potent beta cell toxin', yet the FDA allow Big Food to use it. The link between alloxan and diabetes is as crystal clear as the link between cholesterol and heart disease. Scientists have known of the alloxan-diabetes connection for years.

AP white flour, nutritionally comatose after devitalizing industrial-strength processing, contains neither heavenly nutrients nor fiber. The gazillions of tasty brand name flour products oozing across the floor of America's food culture rapidly convert to sugar inside your Temple, have high glycemic indices, contribute to degenerative diseases, and plump your trunk. White bread's glycemic index is 72, while table sugar's index is 59. No "Wonder" the pancreas must pump out so much insulin, which in time, leads to insulin resistance and pancreatic exhaustion, causing blood sugar to rise, leading to type II diabetes. White bread, bagels, croissants, biscuits, pasta, bread sticks, cookies and cakes, pie and pizza crust, have a high glycemic index. They break down into glucose spiking blood sugar. Therefore eating them could aggravate diabetes and fertilize the disease of obesity.

Whole grains don't throw your Temple into a sugar-fueled drug-like dependency cycle. Replace white flour pasta with Barilla Plus, Barilla Gluten-free, or rice and quinoa versions. Replace AP flour products with rice, potato flour or robust artisan whole grain flours, or Ezekiel and Rudi's Bakery goods. Whole grain food fare brims with colon- cleansing fiber, digests slower so you feel fuller longer and end up eating less, and you'll intake more health-giving nutrients. Healthier carbs should come from fresh, unadulterated gifts of earth such as apples, apricots, bananas, cantaloupe, peaches, pears, oranges, figs, grapes, kiwi, pineapples, plums, strawberries, blueberries, dates, raisins, legumes, dried peas, peanuts, brown rice, bulgur, wheat berries, oatmeal, rye, and quinoa. After 30 days, if you don't feel mental, spiritually, and physically better, have improved blood glucose readings, sue me. But, I'm sure you'll thank me instead.

JAMA says simply switching from white flour to oat, quinoa, brown rice, spelt, buckwheat, garbanzo, coconut or rye flours can lower heart disease risk by 20 percent. You deserve the best, dear friends. Awaken, open your minds and grab a fork full of wholesome reality. Even lab rats resist eating white flour.

62
Oil's Well that Ends Well

"Captain, it's reckless homicide, EFA deficiency," blurted the C.S.I. probie as he watched the EMTs load the blue-faced corpse onto the creaking gurney. This was the perp's second heart attack. This time the murderers finished the job. Greg won't be showing up tonight to walk the dog or have a happy family supper.

The captain pondered the tragedy. The triggerman: hydrogenated oil, aka trans fats saturating grocery store and restaurant ingredients. The COD: heart disease from eating hydrogenated oils plus a diet devoid of essential fatty acid (EFA's) Omega 3 and a lifetime of sucking down dead food our Creator hadn't intended us to eat. The low-fat diet hoopla stripped America's food supply of EFA's triggering a crime wave of diseases. His heart sank when he read children brought up on low fat diets without EFA's are more likely to be sickly and frequently exhibit aggressive behavioral problems and learning debilities. Big Food knows low-fat foods have much longer shelf lives than fatty foods so they've hired advertisers to create fat-phobia. He learned corporations take perfectly healthy raw oils, in their God-given state, chemically extracted them, exposed them to soda ash, and then de-gum, refine, neutralize, filter, bleach, deodorized, and heat to very high temperatures. Pick up some junk food, read the ingredient label and you'll see the term "hydrogenated."

Later the captain got online to profile hydrogenated oils. His moral curiosity wanted to know how the FDA could approve such claptrap. His eye caught an intriguing web site on the health benefits of Omega 3. "Wow, they actually heal!" The Temple requires Omega 3's for life and health but cannot make it from anything else we eat; therefore, it must be obtained from food. "Essential" meaning too little for too long shortens lives. Grind up EFA-rich flax or chia seeds in a coffee grinder then sprinkle them on everything you eat. Cold-water fish eaten twice a week should supply you with enough, but I understand salmon farms put food coloring and antibiotics in the feed.

Every cell, tissue, gland and organ in our body requires EFA's. Nutritionally illiterate doctors won't tell you your heart attack, stroke or embolism was caused by EFA deficiency, or that your arthritis, depression, diabetes, weak bones, dry skin, low energy, bipolar, obsessive-compulsive, anxiety, hormone imbalance, or poor healing can be signs of insufficient Omega-3 in the diet. Grocery store and whole foods grocers carry a delicious rainbow of healthful, environmentally friendly cooking oil and junk food alternatives. Politely ask questions and look around ankle level. That's where you'll find the delicately fragrant expeller, cold pressed olive, unrefined coconut, and nut oils brimming with fats that heal.

The next morning over oatmeal with blueberries, and hot tea, our captain poured over the evidence. The Cleveland Clinic and the American Dietetic Association say, "In the body, hydrogenated oils act like saturated fats and tend to raise blood cholesterol levels. Be prudent how much you consume, especially if you have high cholesterol levels already." Health experts agree, after several decades of research, consumption of hydrogenated oil promotes heart disease, strokes, cancer, diabetes, immune dysfunction, obesity, and reproductive problems. Up against the wall and spread 'em'!

63
Grab a Spear, My Dear or/ Asparagus Tips

As pudgy Robins sing and the gray mood of winter lifts, Mother Nature's ultimate finger food, asparagus, pokes its purple tips through the warming soil. I recall Mom cautioning my brothers and me as we fantasized asparagus spears as swords in our Erol Flynn-esque swashbuckling backyard fantasy, "Don't run with the asparagus, you'll poke someone's eye out!" Aw, Maw!

Since ancient times this member of the lily family was reserved for royalty and rulers. Its name is derived from the Greek word, *asparago,* meaning to "sprout" or "shoot up". The Egyptians cultivate it and Romans from Pliny, to Julius Caesar horded the wild spear, evidence of Hippocrates proclamation of food as medicine. Ancient Chinese herbalists have used asparagus root for centuries.

Five crisp, green ounces provide 60 percent of the recommended daily allowance for folacin required for blood cell growth, the prevention of liver disease, cervical cancer, colon and rectal cancer, and heart disease. The king of vegetables contains steroidal glycosides, which have anti-inflammatory properties to ease the pain of arthritis. Inflammation's been profoundly linked to heart disease and many of today's largely-preventable diseases.

Asparagus contains potassium which helps regulate cellular electrolyte balance within cells and maintains heart functions and blood pressure. It explodes with fiber, thiamin, B6, K, and the Rutin that fortifies your Holy Temple's capillary walls. It's rich in antioxidant vitamins A, C, and E, and a mild diuretic. The green sensation contains glutathione that helps cells break down toxic environmental contaminants that destroying DNA. Glutathione repairs DNA, stimulates immune function. That's what Hippocrates was talking about, food as mouthwatering medicine.

A word of caution for those who take the blood thinner Coumadin / Warfarin to prevent blood clots. Vitamin K in asparagus promotes bone health and triggers blood clotting but alters Pro-Time / INR numbers. Always check with your phlebotomist, but please, don't stop eating green veggies. Instead, work with your phlebotomist and adjust your warfarin to your heavenly green diet.

Asparagus' delicious, cosmic healing mojo is diminished by over-cooking; raw is infinitely best. I know that's a stretch for you, but try. You can do it. Or, steam it for one minute. "As quick as cooking asparagus" was a Roman saying meaning something had to be accomplished rapidly. To steam, place washed, whole trimmed asparagus on a steamer rack over rapidly boiling water. Cover and begin timing. BTW: mushy canned asparagus is nutritionally DOA plus, cans contain cancerous BPA. Lots of toxins loiter in our food supply, dear readers. Caveat Emptor.

Asparagus can be steamed, sautéed in olive oil or rub the spears with a little olive oil, dust with sea salt and pepper then grill on two sides for no more than 2 minutes. Prior to service, trickle fresh lemon juice on the spears for flattering flavor and restorative glutathione. At home, Sandi and I sauté small pieces of asparagus for a brief moment, then we add whipped egg whites to make a wonderful scramble. Add some low fat cheese, but don't go nuts with it. There is life without "Yellow Gravy" a.k.a. Hollandaise sauce or commercial butter. You can live without it...and a lot longer, I might add. Try local butter from happy, grass-fed cows.

Over-cooking deserves a good flogging. Instantly after brief blanching, "shock" the verdant gems in an ice water bath to stop the cooking and maintain brilliant green color. After cooking, if your asparagus has gone limp, you've blown it.

And finally, if after eating asparagus, you are one of the 40% of the population whose urine smells like pungent rotten eggs or cooking cabbage, you're okay; nothing died within your innards. It's caused by the sulfur compounds in the magical vegetable. So don't freak out and use this as a lame excuse not to eat healing asparagus. Celebrate the joyous arrival of spring by embracing the healing, restorative green gift of our generous, loving Creator.

64
Digestion and Your Inner Wilderness

If you've viewed my weekly CBS segment, then you know a bell rings when we say "fiber." If you're one of the dying culture of meat and 'tater eaters, chances are your fiber-starved colon's backed-up, your tummy bloated and you're farting a lot while old food dawdling in your odiferous inner environment stagnates.

Most folks have up to 15 pounds of old, dried, and decaying poo loitering in their fiber-less colons causing autointoxication. These are poisons and waste that, via the help of living foods, could be swept from your colon, but instead, are reabsorbed into your vegaphobic bloodstream. Environmental toxins accumulate in the Temple via air, water, food or contact with skin. Every earthling is toxic from today's industrialized world. Small daily exposures from breakfast cereal, toothpaste, shampoo, soap, perfume, deodorant, hair dye, newspapers, magazines, exhaust fumes, new carpet and new mattresses, dry cleaning or a newly-painted bedroom will increasingly accumulate, exceed and even incapacitate our Temple's ethereal ability to purify it.

Would you know if you were achieving less than your potential? Got fatigue, brain fog, constipation, or yeast infections? Do you need Roto-Rooter or a powerful garden hose? Then it's time to thoroughly cleanse, unblock, and restore your internal ecosystem's balance of good and bad bugs. Once you rid your environment of the accrued waste build-up, you'll feel lighter, younger, and cleaner after toxins finally exit the dark caves and crevasses of your inner wilderness. Sorry, Exlax or a colonoscopy doesn't count. However, a glass of warm prune juice rocks in emergencies. I call it a depth charge.

By following simple dietary guidelines, your colon will regularly and in a timely manner flow like a river in spring, releasing the dam of damaging toxins. When it comes to detoxing your Holy Temple, there are many techniques and supplements you can take, but the best way is eating lots of these heavenly foods that stimulate your Temple to detox, just as our benevolent Creator planned. Eat gobs of easy-to-digest raw fresh fruits and vegetables, green plant foods, nuts and seeds, legumes, oily cold water fish with Omega 3, lemons, limes, oranges and garlic and drink plenty of green tea and water. My favorite depth-charge is two tablespoons of ground flax seed in my daily fruit and veggie smoothie.

Take antioxidants and a food-based multi-vitamin-mineral supplement routinely. Ever hear of Kombucha tea? Drinking probiotic Kombucha promotes good health and helps millions of people with its excellent detoxifying and immune-enhancing assets. There are no known negative reactions from drinking Kombucha tea, except for when it's improperly brewed. Stick with a mainstream brand found at most community health food stores. It does however, contain about 1% alcohol. Beer is 3.5 to 6. Its origins are lost in history, but in early records 2,000 years ago it was known as "the elixir of long life". After an antibiotic regimen, drink a bottle of fizzy, living Kombucha to restore peace in the valley, or your inner universe will be whacked out for months. Hollywood celebrities and movers and shakers swear by the ancient fermented beverage found at farmers' markets, grocery store, and health food stores. It has friendly probiotic bugs found in yogurt, but billions more. Silly Activa is for the unaware and a waste of money. Probiotics, pro-life, can also be purchased in the refrigerator section of your vitamin shop.

It's about loving yourself so much that you don't want to make yourself suffer anymore. You clean your home, garage and car interior, so why not your sacred Temple. It requires the conscious daily intake and symbiosis of fresh, living foods, fibrous foods, and friendly bugs which will help to cleanse, get things moving, and restore your natural GI balance. It'll be a moving experience. You're beautiful and worth it!

65
Your Cells' Major Players

We're held together by roughly 100 trillion, cooperating, vibrating cells, each containing 10,000 more molecules than the Milky Way has stars ... all working in synchronicity; permitting us to achieve our highest potential. But, only if supported. Your Temple, when fed the proper building blocks, is infinitely more powerful than you've been led to believe.

For this to happen, cells require daily intakes of 40 basic nutrients absorbed from a variety of plant foods. To be sure you're getting the daily recommendation; eat a well-balanced diet born from nature, not a Chinese factory, including a food-based, multi-vitamin with trace minerals.

Protein plays a huge role in cell growth and cell damage repair. Most Americans inhale way too much protein, but a deficiency results in problems with your skin, hair, nails, blood, organs and muscles. Protein comes from beef, chicken, fish, pork, local eggs and low-fat dairy. Plant foods like beans, greens, nuts, tempeh, grains and seeds contain protein. Protein intake should be 10 to 35 percent of your daily calories, according to the

USDA's Dietary Guidelines for Americans 2010. For a 2,000-calorie diet, this equates to 50 to 175 g of protein daily.

Iron builds red blood cells. A deficiency could result in weakness or fatigue, aka, anemia. Foods rich in iron include beans, beef, chicken, shrimp, peas, dried fruit, potatoes, spinach, whole grains and tomato juice. Adult women need 18 mg of iron each day, while older women and men should shoot for 8 mg daily. If you are pregnant or breastfeeding, check with your pediatrician.

Vitamin B-12 supports formation of new red blood cells and is only found in animal foods. If you're a vegan or vegetarian, please supplement with a B-Complex that includes B-12. Adults need 2.4 mcg of this B vitamin each day to support healthy blood cells.

Antioxidants fight snarky free radical damage from exposure to environmental toxins and a poor diet that increase risk for cancer and heart disease. Fruits and vegetables are superb sources of antioxidants which lower the occurrence of these diseases. Antioxidants are in dark chocolate, cacao chocolate, red wine, beans, whole grains and fish. A well-balanced dose of antioxidants support healthy cells in all parts of your Temple.

Folic acid, vitamin B6, riboflavin and thiamin are important to t-cells and their quantity. T-cells are white blood cells that protect your Temple against infection. Foods rich in vitamins and minerals are essential to keeping t-cell count up. The best way to get a maximum amount of these nutrients: eat lots of Farmer's market summer fruits and vegetables. Dark green leafy vegetables, cauliflower, broccoli, squash, tomatoes, strawberries and carrots are all nutrient- rich produce that may increase t-cells.

The infinite universe provides everything we need to return to our original, beautiful wholeness. Each cell nucleus holds the miraculous blueprint to create, sustain, restore, and repair the whole--the intelligence of the universe. You are a beautiful, worthy miracle.

66
A Fishy Kettle of Catch-22

While health specialists urge Americans to eat more Omega 3 cold water fish, simultaneously, marine scientists caution farm raised, grocery fish are drowning in ungodly pollutants, preserved with carbon monoxide, and contain precious little Omega 3 essential fatty acids (EFA's). Some types of fish may contain high levels of mercury, PCBs (polychlorinated biphenyls), dioxins and other environmental contaminants. Levels of these substances are generally highest in older, larger, predatory fish and marine mammals. If you can't afford fresh caught Alaskan Salmon, and who can, cast your nets for flax, chia seed and nuts.

Remember the studies revealing Inuit Eskimos had low rates of heart disease despite their diet of lip-smacking whale blubber and oily fish? Turns out omega-3's in the fish protected the garden-less Eskimo health. Omega-3's, EPA and DHA are in oily, fatty, cold water fish such as salmon, mackerel, krill, sardines, herring, seals, whales and supplements. EFA's are indispensable components in normal, healthy cell structure, and help protect your Temple's heart and vascular system. A 1998 JAMA study of over 20,000 individuals discovered eating two servings of fish per week reduced mortality risk from sudden cardiac events by 40 percent.

However, a report was published in the May 9, 2013 issue of the New England Journal of Medicine with one expert saying the evidence on omega-3 fatty acids has been mixed. "Some prior clinical trials have shown a beneficial effect of omega-3 fatty acids derived from fish -- also known as fish oil or n-3 polyunsaturated fatty acids -- in patients with established cardiovascular disease or to prevent cardiovascular events in the general adult population," said Dr. Gregg Fonarow, a professor of cardiology at UCLA. "However, other clinical trials have shown no benefit." Based on the totality of current evidence, the pendulum appears to be shifting away from omega-3 fatty acid supplementation providing significant cardiovascular event reduction," Fonarow said. There is nothing quite like eating the real, wild-caught thing, however. Do the best you can. Ecologically disastrous Fukushima contaminated most northern Pacific fishing waters, and the real truth we won't like to hear, has yet to surface.

With the soaring cost of our aquatic edibles, increasing popularity of plant-based diets, fears about mercury, food dyes, carbon monoxide, antibiotics, and PCB's in seafood, awakened populations are pursuing alternative EFA's sources for defense against Alzheimer's to decrease HDL and increase LDL, lower pesky triglycerides, and prevent blood clotting. Now you know why they're "essential". Reel in your line! The reality: the EPA reports Earth's sacred rivers, lakes, streams, estuaries, mangroves, swamps and Mother Ocean are contaminated and becoming precariously acidic. Fish are sodden with hundreds of cancerous, environmental and agribusiness chemical substances not designed to enter the Holy Temple. Factory fish farms are nasty gulags pumped with antibiotics and irreverent Agrichemical run-off; not what our loving God envisioned. Plus they're fed cheap soy and corn by-products (corn & soy?) and factory farm slaughterhouse beef (beef?) byproducts. The sweet, gentle giants are ruminant grass eating vegetarians by divine design, not corn-eating cannibals. New studies expose seafood may be mislabeled 25 to 70 percent of the time. What you seek may not be what you get. According to FDA port inspectors, a third of seafood sold in the U.S. is mislabeled as one type when it's actually something cheaper. "Don't that make your brown eyes blue?"

Not nourished by their celestially assigned native diet, they're fed orange dye-pills so the flesh will appear orange. Consequently, natural omega-3 from farmed fish is belly-up due to the abnormal diet man thrust upon the captive aquatic critters. Clearly, we're crappy stewards of creation. Man tweaks laws of the universe for consumerist convenience.

In 650 BC, Hippocrates wrote about flax relieving abdominal pain. About the same era, Theophrastus recommended flax mucilage as a cough remedy. During the 8th Century, Charlemagne considered flax so important for the health of his subjects he passed laws and regulations requiring its consumption. Flax seeds are extremely hard, making them difficult to crack. Grind up the shiny brown seeds in a coffee grinder to unleash the golden Omega oil. Chia seed stands alone and needs no grinding. Need more colon cleansing fiber? Add ground flax or chia seed to any dish and things will come out you ate long, long ago. Fibrous cha-cha Chia seed, a complete protein, is the highest plant source of Omega-3 on earth. If you are vegetarian or allergic to seafood, consider green leafy vegetables, almonds, pine nuts, walnuts, ground flax seeds or their oil, but not soybeans, tofu or canola oil. Avoid sugar-coated or salted nut varieties. Walnuts are a high-calorie protein, so use them to replace less healthy proteins, such as cheese and red meat.

Even in the golden years of life's journey, you can still benefit from re-learning how to eat, proper stewardship and by cultivating positive habits which allow Heaven's food to nourish cells, rather than chemically taint them. Your Temple is strong, worthy and beautiful. Celebrate health. From fish, plant, seed, or supplement, EFA's are indispensable.

67
Alzheimer's Disease and Food

Like a scene from an amnesiac horror movie, I'm freaking out at the proposition of waking up, looking over at my loving wife of 23 years, emitting a Homer Simpson shriek asking "Who are you? Why are you in my bed?" The privilege of cooking and nourishing Sandi is an expression of my love and respect for her. Since I cook every meal we eat, I'm responsible for Sandi's physical and mental health and ultimate wellbeing.

What you eat is far more responsible for creating health than you've been led to believe. Preventing, managing and reversing Alzheimer's intensity is largely under your control. Yes, it's often genes but It's also in our lifestyle choices. Alzheimer's disease is a progressive, degenerative disorder that attacks the brain's nerve cells, or neurons, resulting in loss of memory, thinking, language skills, and behavioral changes. It is not a natural part of aging as we're misled. The Alzheimer's Association of America (AAA) says there is no cure. Common behavioral changes include sleep disturbances, physical or verbal outbursts, emotional distress, restlessness, pacing, shredding paper or tissue, delusions and hallucinations. Other identified risk factors include high blood pressure, coronary heart disease, and diabetes. Women are more at risk for developing Alzheimer's. It's estimated 10% of the population over 65 years of age have Alzheimer's, and 50% over 80 have some level of the disease. There are currently over 5 million Americans with Alzheimer's and that's predicted to grow to nearly 15 million by 2050.

Give your Temple tools to defend and protect itself. Eating from the current American food system does absolutely nothing to advance and sustain your Temple's health. The Alzheimer's disease brain is under significant oxidative stress. The AMA's Archives of Neurology and Psychiatry suggests the right combination of foods is "one of the most important modifiable environmental factors" that could reduce individual risk of Alzheimer's disease. Finding simple ways to reduce the risk of developing Alzheimer's disease could be as easy as eating the right combination of "anti-Inflammatory" foods, including antioxidants and vitamin E and a 1:1 ratio of essential omega 3 and omega 6 fatty acids found in fish, poultry, nuts, and fruits and vegetables. Evidence indicates diets low in omega-3 fats and high in omega-6 fats promote Alzheimer's disease; antioxidant-rich diets may also reduce risk and severity. Currently, Americans eat a disproportionate ratio of 23 to 1 favoring omega 6 and, that's a big health problem. Research discovered omega 6 counteracts omega 3 efficacy. Omega 6 is in of oils like peanut, corn, peanut, soybean, walnut or safflower, as well as mayonnaise, crackers and chips, cookies, pies, cakes, and salad dressings. Too much Omega 6 contributes to Alzheimer's. Prevention is infinitely the best strategy.

68
The Great Fluoride Con-troversy

Toothpaste: "WARNING: Keep out of reach of children under 6 years of age. If you accidentally swallow more than used for brushing, seek PROFESSIONAL HELP or contact a POISON CONTROL center immediately."

A crushing body of evidence and the raised eyebrow of the FDA incriminate Fluoride in toothpaste and mouthwash as a toxic drug "NOT FIT FOR HUMAN CONSUMPTION".

Breaking Fox News: "EPA Reverses Itself on Fluoride." Unaware there's a problem? That happens when folks blindly trust, don't question authority, and live in blissful ignorance. For decades fluoride's been marketed as obligatory for oral hygiene. It's in most toothpastes and mouthwashes while parents are aggressively encouraged to give their kids fluoride treatments. After all, 9 out of 10 "experts" can't be wrong. *Cue distrust.*

Historically, our leaders have an embarrassingly dreadful track record acknowledging health risks associated with certain corporate chemicals, especially when its agencies have already determined these products as "safe". Sad how times change, but truth does not. It's taken government 60 years to admit Americans have been overexposed to this harmful chemical though several studies by the National Toxicology Program that show fluoride causes bone cancer, particularly in young men. This jives with studies documenting it causes cellular mutations associated with cancer. Drinking fluoridated water causes damage to the brain and kidneys, compromises the sacred pineal gland, trashes immunity, lowers IQ, and in Washington DC specifically, they determined people drinking only one quart from their public water supply each day ingest more than 1,428 times the safe dose of fluoride which explains the current political insanity and ambitious greed in DC.

In 1950, Procter and Gamble tossed 3 million at Indiana University Bloomington bio-chemists to contrive a cavity-preventing prototype. They ran clinical trials on 1500 innocent children and 400 naïve adults. After testing, a good half of the participants showed substantial decrease in dental caries. Viola, Crest was invented. Back in the 40s, our "scholarly" leaders encouraged municipal water authorities to add fluoride to community's drinking water. According to the CDC, approximately 70 percent of the U.S. population ingests fluoride through drinking water; in Europe it's only 10%.

In an encouraging reversal, Fox reported the EPA will lower the maximum amount of fluoride in drinking water because of growing evidence supporting fluoride's snarky effects to children's Temples. In 2006, the National Academy of Sciences reported dental fluorosis, caused by too much fluoride, puts children at risk of developing breakdown of tooth enamel, discoloration and pitting. In addition, other study found excessive ingested fluoride increases the risk of bone fractures and abnormalities.

That's why I lovingly badger you to be vigilant, due diligence and admit "experts" are often dead wrong. Revisit your dental hygiene ritual, read labels, and look for xylitol on the label. A reverse osmosis system removes fluoride.

While brushing your pearly-whites, recall your childhood fluoride treatments. Ever read the dire warning on brand name toothpastes? Without the shadow of a doubt, fluoride should never be consumed. The EPA classifies fluoride as a "chemical having substantial evidence of developmental neurotoxicity." Fluoride's banned in Sweden, Norway, Denmark, Germany, Italy, Belgium, Austria, France, and The Netherlands as the U.S. fluoridates every water supply, coast to coast.

The U.S. Consumer Product Safety Commission say fluorides, hazardous waste from the chemical fertilizer industry, are also in household cleaning solutions for metal, tile, brick, cement, wheels, radiators, siding, toilets, ovens, and drains. Fluorides are also found in rust and water stain removers, silver solder, etching compounds, laundry soap, air conditioner coil cleaners, floor polishes, and oh yes, your toothpaste, and minty mouthwash.

A Scientific American study concluded, "Fluoride can subtly alter endocrine function, especially in the thyroid." Iodine, an essential trace element vital for normal growth and development, controls thyroid function which in turn significantly influences your Temple's metabolic processes. Ugh oh! Fluoride inhibits iodine absorption, ergo; Americans need more iodine which will immediately increases the excretion of bromide, fluoride, chlorine, and some heavy metals including mercury and lead. Iodine supplementation is the best way to increase iodine levels in adults and children whose thyroids are already compromised. We prefer Kelp tablets.

The National Research Council of the National Academies report said, ".... evidence indicates several types of Fluoride alter normal endocrine function." Long-term, low doses of fluoride can cause Hypothyroidism which is at epidemic levels in the U.S.

Feeling disconnected from your higher source? Tragically, your Temples pineal gland, your third eye, connects you with the Divine but attracts the highest concentration of fluoride, causing it to become calcified and useless, rendering you spiritually detached.

Brain Research Journal says fluoride affects your mind by encouraging uptake of aluminum into your brain producing tangles associated with Alzheimer's disease. Chinese studies warned fluoride, at the doses children are now receiving, might be causing IQ and behavioral problems.

GreenMedInfo.com reports that Americans would have better health and a lower incidence of cancer and fibrocystic disease of the breast if they consumed more iodine. Your cells need iodine to regulate their metabolism. Without it, people may suffer from swollen glands in the throat, thyroid diseases, increased fluoride toxicity, decreased fertility rates, increased infant mortality rates, and mental impedance.

Alas, Fluoride, imposed upon us as a treatment for dental disease, cannot be removed from tap water by any other detoxifying method other than reverse osmosis. Scientific evidence over the past 50 years shows that sodium fluoride shortens your life span, promotes various cancers and mental disturbances, and most importantly, makes humans stupid, docile, and obedient, which is all well and good if you're an anti-American terrorist.

If you hold stock in the chemical fertilizer industry, the public water supply shouldn't be a dumping ground of hazardous waste.

*Waldbott, George, MD, Fluoride: The Great Dilemma, 1978, Coronado Press, Lawrence, KS
*Yaimouyiannis, John, Fluoride: The Aging Factor, 1993, Health Action Press, Delaware
*Varner, J A, et al, "Chronic Administration of Aluminum Fluoride or Sodium Fluoride to Rats in Drinking water: Alterations in Neuronal and Cerebrovascular Integrity", Brain Research, 784(1-2):284-298, 1998, 1998, Feb 16.
*Isaacson, R L, et al, "Toxin-Induced Blood Vessel Inclusions Caused By the Chronic Administration of Aluminum and Sodium Fluoride and Their Implications in Dementia", Ann NY Acad Science, 825():152-166, 1997, Oct 15.
*Varner, J A, et al , "Chronic Aluminum Fluoride Administration, Part I: Behavioral Observations", Behavior Neural Biology, 61(3):233-241, 1994, May.
*Burgstahler, A W, Colquhoun, J, "Neurotoxicity of Fluoride", Fluoride, 29:57-58, 1996 and
Li, X S, Zhi, J L, Gao R O, "Effects of Fluoride Exposure on the Intelligence of Children", Fluoride, 28:182-189, 1995 and
Mullenix, P J, et al, "Neurotoxicity of Sodium Fluoride on Rats", Neurotoxicity and Teratology, 17:169-177, 1995 and
*Zhao, L B, et al, "Effect of Fluoridated Water Supply on Children's Intelligence", Fluoride, 29:190-192, 199

69
Teach your children well

Kids' food needs are the same they were 20 years ago. However, the food they eat today is doggie doo, horrid. In fact, science says they cause sterility, obesity and diabetes. 'Lunchables' is a diabolical example. Temptingly marketed, this demon is laden with an un-godly amount of salt, HFCS, bad fats, food colorings, nitrates, wheat and immune-depleting sugar. But, man is it profitable.

Kids' Temples need 40 vitamins and 90 minerals daily. Megavitamins, large doses of vitamins, aren't a good idea for children. To accomplish this, kids need a variety of fresh, chemically-free, nutritious food in its God-given state. Today's fake foods are nutritionally D.O.A., a result of immoral industrial modification.

Kids need whole foods prepared with Mom's nourishing kitchen love. Growing bodies require quality materials to grow big and strong. Prepare wholesome, balanced lunches at home. Are their bag lunches based on your convenience or their needs? It's time for loving parents to update their nutritional know-how and stop projecting their silly fears of food upon their kids. Let them make up their own minds. We're not born to fear fruits and vegetables, we're taught. Time-strapped parents tell me there's no time to prepare healthy lunches. Gimme a break! One child told me her parents give her a "Poop Tart" and a can of Mountain Dew, full of High Fructose Corn Syrup and mercury for breakfast. Sigh. Listen up Mom and Dad: "Poop Tarts" are a form of child abuse.

Harris Polls estimates about 1.4 million American youth are vegetarian, while about three million never eat meat. Vegetarian kids have lower risk of obesity, cancer and heart disease. Give them a kid's multi-vitamin-mineral supplement, too. It's essential offspring get plenty of clean protein, vitamins B12 and D-3, iron, calcium and many other nutrients and minerals most people get from meat, eggs and dairy.

Face the reality: today's children are heavier than ever and face somber, lifetime health consequences. An overweight child is more likely to become an overweight adult. Parents have the greatest influence on their child's diet and exercise habits and make daily decisions that will affect their child's current and future nutrition and health patterns. Parents' mindful responsibility is to teach children to lead healthy lives now and when they're adults. Helping children maintain a healthy weight doesn't have to be a battle. Don't put your child on a 'Fad' diet. Popular with adults, they're not designed for children. A balanced diet is the goal.

Lovingly teach them before unhealthy choices become habits. Explain you'll be making important changes in family meals; eating will be different but fun. Allow sweet treats in mindful moderation rather than eliminate them. Rewarding them with a Snickers bar if they eat their broccoli says candy is more valuable. Be a role model. If you eat right, your children will too. Your beloved kids love, adore and need you. Love them back with healthful role modeling.

70
Dandelions Don't Tell No lies!

You dig and yank; they lurk and bloom bright yellow droplets, not of joy, but of defiance while they seem to say: "*Bwa ha ha!*"

When I see a soothing emerald patchwork of bright, brilliant yellow polka dots I perceive Earth's exquisiteness, nutrition and generosity. Dandelions aren't weeds; they're divine gifts of food as medicine. Today, they're the cockroach of plants, a bane to vanity lawns. Thoreau would freak out. A friend's toddler observed, "Mommy, we are the only ones who love dandelions, everyone else wants to kill them." Mom assured her there are many evolved folks who let dandelions grow and eat them. "Grandpa lived on fried dandelion flowers throughout the depression."

"Mommy, what's the depression?"

Dandelions arrived onboard the Mayflower due to their medicinal benefits. Settlers discovered over 2,000 uses for various green herbs we consider undesirable, bitter lawn pests. Dandelion roots have been used in tonics and cures for centuries, yet today we repel, heartlessly spewing them with toxic Round-Up to 'keep up with the Jones's; gimme a break. What happened to the 10th Commandment? Getting folks to stop using 'MonSatan's' Round-up is like trying to recover dandelion seeds after they're thrown to the wind. Society "blind eyes" the Karmic consequences of murdering God's green gifts. We are stewards, not destroyers of life. Awakened green gardeners refuse to poison the "ugly weed" with chemicals that drain into your invaluable, dwindling watershed, and into your daily food.

Try unsprayed young dandelion greens, boiled potatoes, hard-boiled eggs, red onions, garlic, olive oil and apple cider vinegar. One friend recollects her dad picking them in the spring. The father said eating greens was a spring tonic. He cooked them dipped in flour and fried in butter. At home, Sandi and I put spring leaves into smoothies. We've made tea from the flower and often have fresh dandelions in little vases when they're abundant. When my friend's mother was in the last stages of lymphoma, she'd sit on the porch watching me garden. She heard my neighbor was spraying his dandelions, so she got up with her walker and sat in his yard all day and picked his dandelions. The neighbor came to her funeral and announced he was no longer spraying dandelions.

The slandered miracle food is more nutritious than most vegetables. Unfortunately, many refuse them due to their bitterness. However, "the more bitter, the more better." Like our Creator planned, they heal many ailments: baldness, dandruff, toothache, sores, and fevers, rotting gums, weakness, lethargy and depression. Data from the USDA supports dandelions help relieve many ailments. They have more vitamin A than spinach, more C than tomatoes, plus iron, calcium and potassium. The "cockroach of plants" prevent or cure liver hepatitis or jaundice; act as a tonic and gentle diuretic to purify your blood, cleanse your system, dissolve kidney stones, improve gastro-intestinal health, assist in weight reduction, cleanse your skin and eliminate acne, improve your bowel function, working equally well to relieve both constipation and diarrhea, prevent or lower high blood pressure, prevent or cure anemia, lower your serum cholesterol by as much as half, eliminate or drastically reduce acid indigestion and gas buildup by cutting the heaviness of fatty foods, prevent or cure various forms of cancer, prevent or control diabetes mellitus, and, at the same time, have no negative side effects and selectively act on only what ails your Temple. A divine miracle.

Love your souls' earthly home. Don't use un-holy Round-Up (what, me, guilt you?). Instead pick 'em, wash 'em, eat 'em and feel their healing mojo flow from cell to cell. Blow the pretty dandelion heads, leaving the little ivory colored bald head with tiny holes and eat the serrated leaves in salad. If you have a dog, give the leaves a good washing. If ChemLawn sprays, don't eat them, period! Transcend Dandephobia into love of life, health and reverence for your verdant backyard apothecary.

71
Want to Get Fat? Sweeteners Where it's At

Seems everybody's becoming wary regarding what's in their food. Awakening Americans are discovering foods made by man have proven a folly as obesity and chronic disease rates soar and both IQ and sperm count plummet. Aspartame, AKA

Equal or NutraSweet, the blue packages of death, is an excitoneurotoxic drug linked to brain damage and should be removed from schools and banned from civilization.

NutraSweet contains three neurotoxins: methanol wood alcohol, aspartic acid used as pesticide, and phenylalanine, a brain tumor agent. Certain snakes, scorpions, frogs and fish are known for secreting deadly substances known as neurotoxins.

The black-hearted, multi-billion dollar aspartame industry wants you to believe "aspartame kills" is an urban legend, that you'd have to drink 100 cans of diet soda a day to be harmed by aspartame. That's a black lie. Can you say accumulation? Aspartame was never and cannot be proven to be safe without telling lies. For individuals who are overweight, not only is diet soda not a diet product, but a chemically altered, multiple sodium (salt) and aspartame-containing product that actually makes you crave carbohydrates and gain weight. It contains formaldehyde, or embalming fluid which is stored in the fat cells, particularly in the hips and thighs. The National Soft Drink Association did a 30-page protest in the '80s, mentioning aspartame was unstable, that it depleted serotonin (a substance that tells you to stop eating, you're full) which often triggers a carbohydrate binge. The Atlanta Journal Constitution reported back in 1998, "Aspartame is a Pandora's box of toxins and tumor agents that have 92 FDA acknowledged ways to ruin your life, death being one!" Book 'em, Danno!

Over decades, the FDA has received thousands of complaints (not all of them seem to be accounted for, like erased IRS emails), and by 1996 the FDA admitted to receiving over 10,000 "official" complaints. The FDA has stated that aspartame is the most complained about substance in its history. Dr. Kessler, retired Director of the FDA, has said less than 1 percent of victims actually file a complaint. This balloons those over 10,000 formal complaints to over a million victims who should have filed. Most doctors and victims of aspartame poisoning don't have a clue to the cause of those many painful and expensive problems. Respected Dr. Andrew Weil says everyone should stop using toxic NutraSweet unless stupid is your goal.

Researchers and doctors say aspartame side-effects could take several years to manifest themselves. Among the most frequent symptoms are vision loss, memory loss, obesity, testicular, mammary and brain tumors, seizures, coma, and cancer. Worse still, the symptoms of aspartame poisoning appear to mimic the symptoms of certain major diseases such as fibromyalgia, multiple sclerosis, lupus, ADHD, diabetes, Alzheimer's disease, chronic fatigue, and depression. This makes it very difficult to diagnose.

Read labels. Don't cave to sweet, mindless delusion. Love yourself enough not to put this unholy crap into your Sacred Temple home.

72
We've got to Get Ourselves Back to the Garden

On countless levels, a joyful universal awakening has begun: a shift in social consciousness. It's a foreseen, eagerly anticipated age of enlightenment, peace, love, and understanding. The Age of Aquarius has begun, my friends. The slumbering beast has awakened, experiencing a burning-bush moment. Success ensues when we get out of the way. Mindfully enlightening your green food mentality simply indicates you're learning and growing, the reason for being on this earthly plane.

Even though consumption and super-sizing is the new mantra, Americans have been undernourished for the last 100 years. Disease rates have grown exponentially, paralleled with increased human intake of dead machine cuisine. Post Industrial Revolution food processing practices are at the root of the healthcare catastrophe, not you. To apply blame to this lunacy we only need to face Capitol Hill's good-ol-boys and their obedient Agribusiness lap-dogs. You didn't cause disease rates to soar; they did. It was their uneducated RDA's. Our only blunder is we trusted the soulless information terrorists. Dead, below average food, seasoned with colorfully decorated deception, raw greed and smart-bomb misinformation is enthusiastically endorsed by the deadened FDA. Plus, our "leaders" pat themselves on the back while seeking photo-ops and constituent approval for sending low-grade, nutritionally bankrupt white four with alloxin and arsenic laced rice to distressed Third World countries. However, the "foods" they dispatch are inferior to what's indigenously available to these downtrodden. White rice, AP flour, sugar, succulent military MRE's, valueless canned food with BPA, and canned Spam are all nutritionally insolvent and exacerbate disease, providing little or no sustaining nutrition, just unoccupied calories and self-aggrandizement. Why don't industry cartels simply hold a gun to our heads?

Time's ripe for "green" free-thinkers to confront America's current food Zeitgeist of industrial-strength, almost but not quite edible food-like substances, and then to return to a more preordained, lucid, wholesomely spiritual Locavore approach to eating and living designed by the great Creator. The current limelight on health indicates an admission we've been wrong. However, no one is held culpable in a unique world, circling the proverbial drain.

73
Spring and Rebirth

After dusting off the dreary grayness of winter and savoring spring's first tender greens, consider the infinite universe below the surface of your skin. Often overlooked, your inner ecosystem brims with trillions of needy inhabitants and chemical reactions dependent upon a green, pure, fresh diet, harmonious with our design.

Americans have departed from the path of nutritional righteousness. It's stirring, however to see how swiftly the seed of "Holy Temple ecology" is being reborn within our green consciousness. To restore, give health, and prop up your inner ecology. Your Holy Temple needs to function with efficiency to eliminate the ill health robbing you of the joy of living. Enter Hippocrates, the father of medicine.

The Green Movement focuses on the external world of objects and resources. Though, while "greening" what lies beneath your 1.5 mm of flesh, you need a methodology for compassionately understanding the mechanisms by which it operates. By foraging from earth's universal apothecary, we simultaneously nurture and heal our inner and outer milieu. Consuming a rainbow of sustainable, local foods crammed with vibrating cosmic energy, cultivate, refresh, and strengthen your Holy Temple's mind / body ecosystem like a fresh spring breeze. After considering both and making informed choices, you'll discover local foods are eternally more flavorful, provide more energy, contain vastly more nutrients and make the cooking process a joyful celebration.

There are many disquieting environmental factors affecting gut ecology. Our body intelligence does not recognize alien food not preordained for human consumption. These "foods" and the air you breathe worm their way into digestion. Mono-crop farming causes deficiencies in trace minerals such as zinc and selenium, which aid elimination of toxic elements in food and prop up healthy biological processes. Depletion of nutrients by means of mono-crop agribusiness compromises below-the-skin ecology and the ability to synthesize essential vitamins. Ergo, many are subtly malnourished and susceptible to disease.

Eating without thinking leaves you vulnerable to select foods less healthy for you, the family, and Mother Earth. Mindfully savor the true flavor; think about its source, what it's doing for your viscera, and then express gratitude. Your Temple, in harmonic vibration with the universe, is indeed a miracle you deserve. It's up to your dietary mindfulness. Remember that under the right dietary conditions, your Temple has the inborn ability to heal itself.

74
Recipe for Perfect Health

Food activates your Holy Temple's inner intelligence. The points listed gently and continuously prompt your inner universe, mind, and soul to merge in a joyous flow of intelligence. Once the flow is set up, nothing else is necessary but to enjoy your life and dig crystal clear connection to your oneness.

- Pay attention to eating. Quality triumphs over quantity. Meditate on what's at the end of your fork.

- Pause mindfully before eating and sit in silence – or say grace – so that awareness begins the meal quietly. When eating out, chose quite environments. Hard Rock Café would not be the best choice.
- Think of food as sacred; the family dining table as an altar of gratitude.
- Express gratitude to the universes for its generosity. Prepare and offer the universe a plate of your prepared food.
- Eat when you are hungry and do not eat when you are not. Recognize emotional eating and become stronger by denying it.
- Do not sit down to eat if you are upset – your Holy Temple is better off without food until you calm down and feel better.
- Slow down. Take leisurely time to eat. Chew food well and slowly until it's liquefied. Digestion begins in the mouth.
- Appreciate the company and compliment the hands of the cooked or raw food.
- Avoid eating in any toxic company that makes you feel less than agreeable, but eat with congenial company, non-judgmental friends and family when you can.
- Tell a joke. Laugh. Share a positive story. Hug the ones you're with and then kindly express your love and gratitude for them and everything.

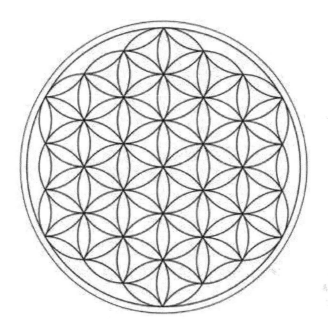

Recipes

Breakfast

Grand Master Breakfast or Dessert Parfait

Here's a breakfast that beautifies the skin, removes toxins, and helps get rid of those unattractive cottage cheese thighs.

- Yogurt fills your bowels with probiotics that help break down nutrients, encourage regularity and allow your skin to maximize the foods you consume
- Bulk from the bran gleans away waste from the bowels and promotes bowel health
- Bran aids in the removal of cholesterol from the blood. Excess circulating cholesterol can lead to bumpy, rough skin and clogged pores. Thus, controlling your cholesterol level can result in smoother skin
- Apples deliver moisture and more fiber to colon which again supports regularity
- Collectively, this dessert promotes beautiful skin by aiding in the efficient removal of toxins from the body while helping the skin retain an optimal moisture level

½ cup of plain, organic yogurt-calcium (Look for coconut milk yogurt, it's the best!)
1/3 cup of all-bran cereal or granola
1 medium apple sliced into cubes
Blueberries-washed thoroughly
60% cacao grated dark chocolate
1 pkg. Stevia (Not Truvia or Stevia in the Raw)
1 Tbsp. ground flax seeds - Omega 3

- In a bowl, add the cubed apples and top with the bran cereal. Top the bran with the low-fat yogurt.
- Swirl in the grated chocolate and the packet of stevia to add a bit of sweetness to this treat. Now top with blueberries, flax, and walnuts.

Apple Cider Oatmeal with Omega 3 Walnuts and Berries
2 Portions
The finest Oatmeal gruel you'll eat!

Our friends at the FDA say oatmeal may reduce cholesterol in the human body. By Using fresh apple cider and not water, the flavor of the oatmeal is ethereal, the blueberries are powerful antioxidants, and the cranberries help prevent bladder infections. Cranberries contain proanthocyanidins (PACs) that can prevent the adhesion of certain bacteria, including *E. coli*, associated with urinary tract infections to the urinary tract wall. The anti-adhesion properties of cranberry may also inhibit the bacteria associated with gum disease and stomach ulcers: http://www.cranberryinstitute.org/healthresearch.htm.

Oatmeal is good for reducing cholesterol, but not the crappy Quaker species. Quaker is excessively processed just like instant white rice. This porridge with the fresh berries and nuts supplies you with Omega 3 essential fatty acids and powerful antioxidant protection. They slow down the aging process, reduce cavities, and the granddaddy of them all...cancer.

Steel cut oats—follow the package instructions (No Instant Quaker or little pre-portioned packages please!)
Fresh organic apple cider
1/2 cup fresh cranberries, washed
1/2 cup fresh or frozen blueberries, washed
1/2 cup walnut pieces
1 tsp. cinnamon
REAL maple syrup to sweeten
1 tsp. of ground flax or Chia seeds for fiber
2 Tbsp. organic unrefined coconut oil
Pinch of sea salt
1 wooden spoon

- In a sauté pan, place the fresh cranberries in the bottom of a sauté pan.
- Next add about 2 tablespoons of maple syrup, apple cider, cinnamon and simmer over LOW heat till you hear the first POP! of

a cranberry.
- Immediately add the oats and coconut oil, stirring continuously with a wooden spoon until the oats absorb the delicious apple flavor and are cooked. Gravity happens and the porridge can scorch easily.
- Add a pinch of sea salt to taste.
- When desired consistency is achieved, pull it off the fire and serve topped with walnut pieces, ground flax, blueberries and cranberries. An irresistible flavor and fibrous bonanza.

Blueberry Whole Grain Pancakes

Mix in medium bowl:
2 cups organic whole wheat or gluten-free flour
2 Tbsp. wheat germ or chia seed
2 tsp. non-aluminum baking powder
½ Cup chopped walnuts or almonds

Beat In:
2 cups organic almond or coconut milk
2 local organic eggs; or the equivalent of 3 egg whites
1 Tbsp. cold-pressed vegetable oil

Stir In:
1 ½ cups washed fresh blueberries
1 cup of walnut pieces

- Lightly oil a frying pan and spoon batter onto a warm pan.
- Cook pancakes as you would normally.

Flourless Pumpkin Pancakes w/Homemade Blueberry Syrup
(Gluten-free)

It's not so easy being gluten-free. Not only is gluten found in grains like wheat, barley, oats and rye, it's also added to many foods as a thickening agent. For example, some ice creams and even ketchup contain gluten. The simple solution: avoid wheat products and processed foods made with processed wheat.

At home, Sandi and I prepare these fiberlicious, healthy and wheat-free pancakes for the family. If you're discreet and don't shine a floodlight on the change, no one will notice because they taste so darned good. Recently we've begun adding organic pumpkin puree and ground flax seed to goose up the nutrition, fiber and Omega 3 essential fatty acids.

Please avoid Aunt Jemima Pancake mix as she's mostly, gag, high fructose corn syrup. The pancake dry-mix brims with aluminum anti-caking agents, refined white flour (the villain) and the "syrup" is composed of vile high fructose corn syrup and yummy artificial flavorings. Opt for the real thing. You and your loved ones deserve the best. Instead of artery detonating butter, try Smart Balance Omega 3 fortified butter substitutes.

Gluten-Free Pancake Mix (Bob's Red Mill & Hodgson Mills @ grocery)
4 local organic egg whites
1/3 cup pumpkin puree
2 Tbsp. ground flaxseed meal (use a coffee grinder)
½ cup chopped walnuts
½ tsp. "real" vanilla extract
1 tsp. cinnamon and a pinch of nutmeg

- Whisk the egg whites till lightly frothy.
- Warm up the skillet or griddle to medium high heat.
- Per instructions, in a large bowl, mix spices and incorporate together with a wire whisk.
- Work in the egg whites, pumpkin puree, flax, walnuts and vanilla.
- Lightly spray a griddle or pan and cook at medium heat.
- Flip them only once when you see the first tiny bubbles form.
- While the pancakes are browning, over low heat, gently warm the "real" maple syrup. Shut off the heat before it comes to a boil

then add 1 cup of fresh or frozen blueberries.
Set aside.
- Serve immediately topped with your fresh, homemade blueberry syrup.

Vegetarian Breakfast Burrito

Vegetarian breakfast burritos make for a fun breakfast and kids love them too. This basic recipe with eggs, salsa and cheese is very simple so you can always add extra spices or seasonal vegetables or whatever turns you on. This recipe is just for one vegetarian breakfast burrito.

2 local organic eggs or egg replacer
2 Tbsp. Almond milk
Sea salt and pepper to taste
1 Tbsp. expeller-pressed vegetable oil, butter from grass-fed cows, coconut oil, or vegan margarine
1/4 cup grated non-cheddar or vegan cheese
2 Tbsp. salsa
1 gluten-free tortilla
1 Tbsp. ground flax seeds

- In a small bowl, whisk the eggs together with the milk until well beaten and season with salt and pepper.
- Heat the oil or butter in a skillet or frying pan over medium-high heat. Carefully add the eggs. Cook, mixing frequently, until you have scrambled eggs of the desired consistency.
- Sprinkle on the flax seed at the end to boost fiber and Omega 3.

Warm the flour tortilla in the microwave for a few seconds just until warm and soft. Place the scrambled eggs in the center of the flour tortilla, and top with cheese and salsa. Wrap and enjoy your vegetarian breakfast burrito!

Nutty Cinnamon Quinoa Porridge

1 cup organic 1% milk or almond milk
1 cup water or apple cider in season
1 cup organic quinoa, rinsed
2 cups fresh black or blueberries
½ tsp. ground cinnamon
1/3 cup chopped pecans
4 tsp. maple syrup (no fraudulent Aunt Jemima, please!)

- Combine milk or cider, water and quinoa in medium saucepan. Bring to boil over high heat. Reduce heat to medium-low; cover and simmer 15 minutes or until most of the liquid is absorbed.
- Turn off the heat; let stand covered 5 minutes. Stir in berries and cinnamon; transfer to four bowls and top with pecans.
- Drizzle each bowl with 1 Tbsp. maple syrup.

Peanut Butter, Berries, Granola and Fruit Breakfast Wraps

4-8 inch fat-free whole wheat tortilla shells (8-9 inches)
½ cup peanut or almond butter
¼ cup fork-crushed strawberries, or your favorite 'All-Fruit' spread
2 medium bananas
¼ cup granola (No Kashi, Pillsbury, or General Mills)

- Spread tortillas with peanut butter, then the spreadable fruit.
- Top with bananas.
- Sprinkle with granola
- Roll up those bad boys.

Spinach and Egg Breakfast Wrap with Avocado and Pepper Jack Cheese

(5-ounce) Box or bag baby spinach, washed and chopped
4 eggs
4 egg whites
1/2 tsp. sea salt-trace minerals

1/4 tsp. pepper
4 ounces shredded pepper jack cheese
1 avocado, sliced-healthiest food on earth
4 Udi's gluten-free tortillas
Hot sauce

- Spray a nonstick skillet over medium-high heat.
- Add spinach and cook, stirring, until wilted, 2 minutes.
- Whisk together eggs and egg whites in a small bowl. Add eggs to skillet and cook, stirring, until cooked through, 3–4 minutes.
- Season with salt and pepper.
- Place 1/4 of egg mixture in the center of each tortilla, and sprinkle with 1 ounce cheese.
- Top with 4 slices avocado and fold, burrito-style. Slice in half and serve.

Smoothies: Functional "Living" Beverages

People would rather swallow than chew. Smoothies, as opposed to Juicing, provide magnificent, fibrous, living bulk nutrition for breakfast, lunch or dinner. Digestion begins in the mouth, so be sure to chew your smoothies so the glands in your mouth can secrete digestive enzymes.

Basic Raw Fruit and Vegetable Smoothie Template

A daily smoothie is an efficient means to insure your Holy Temple is supplied with the required amount of quality sun-kissed fruits and vegetables. "Candied" smoothies purchased at malls and airports are most often sweetened with simple syrup or High Fructose Corn Syrup; AKA, "Fat Fertilizer". Nefarious HFCS is as villainous as sugar, so do not listen to the propaganda set forth by the knuckle draggers from corn industry. It's corn porn. *"Brown-Chickie Brown cow"*. Dust off your blender and it will serve you well. Add ice when needed. However, room temperature food is much easier for your Holy Temple to digest.

The liquid base can be:
Filtered water
Fresh orange juice
Apple cider

Guava or apricot nectar
Cranberry or grape juice
Tomato juice from a jar or homemade
Coconut water or milk
Cashew or almond milk
Never use dairy

Other content options:

Banana, mango, strawberries, blueberries, pears, unpeeled carrot, kale, arugula, avocado, beets and beet greens, ginger, kale, sweet potato chunks, cucumber, silken organic tofu, virgin coconut oil, kiwi, blueberries, ground flax seeds, nut butters, flax seed oil, watermelon, oranges, pineapple, cranberries, lime juice, brewer's yeast, Spirulina, liquid minerals and vitamins, and the list could endlessly go on. I think you get the picture; anything goes. Do not add any dairy to a smoothie with citrus, however. The ensuing curdling stimulated when the citric acid meets dairy in the stomach, strains the digestive process, ergo, accelerating the aging process.

Feelin' Groovy Ginger Pear Smoothie
A perfect breakfast, snack, or light meal

1 chopped pear with skin, washed
3-4 large kale leaves or 2 cups baby spinach
½ inch fresh ginger
2-3 Tbsp. hemp, flax, or chia seeds
1 Tbsp. maple syrup or ½ tsp. stevia powder
2 cups filtered water

- Wash pears, ginger, and kale. Rinse and drain.
- Simply blend all ingredients until smooth – be patient.

Mango and Fig Smoothie

6 dried raw, pitted figs
½ cup warm water
3 ½ oz. silken, organic tofu
3 ½ cups peeled, cubed mango

¾ cup almond milk
1 Tbsp. almond butter
1 Tbsp. local raw honey
1 tsp. ground flax seeds

- Soak figs in warm water for 30 minutes. Drain.
- Place figs in blender; add tofu, almond milk, mango, almond butter, honey, and flax.
- Blend well.
-

Super-Smoothie

1 cup coconut milk
1 avocado
2 bananas
5-10 dates, pitted
Handful pumpkin seeds
2 tsp. powdered Spirulina (can be replaced by a handful of fresh greens if preferred)

- Soak pumpkin seeds overnight and the dates for at least an hour in warm water. Drain.
- Blend the seeds and dates first with a little of the coconut milk before adding all of the other ingredients.
- Sweeten with a smidge of raw honey or other acceptable natural sweetener.

Breakfast Protein Jackpot Smoothie

½ cup raw or regular tahini
½ cup plain organic goat, coconut, or dairy yogurt
½ cup rolled oats
2 Tbsp. raw local honey
½ cup filtered water

- Blend everything until smooth.

Audrey's Chocolate – Coconut –Banana Bliss Smoothie
Serves 1

½ cup fresh coconut water
¼ cup fresh young coconut meat
1 Ripe banana (use peeled/frozen banana for a frozen smoothie)
½ cup fresh purified water
2 Tbsp. carob powder
1 Tbsp. raw cacao (or organic cocoa powder)
1 tsp. fresh ground cinnamon
1 tsp. mesquite powder (optional)
1 tsp. Vita-Mineral Green or other green powder (optional)

- To make this RAW/Living smoothie, put all ingredients in high-speed blender and start blending on low speed and slowly turn to high speed. Blend until thoroughly mixed.

Beet-Carrot-Fennel-Basil Smoothie

1 large beet
3 carrots
1 large handful basil
½ rib fennel

- Wash produce, run through your blender or Vita-mix and enjoy.

A Jar of Pumpkin and Pecan Pie Smoothie

1 frozen banana
1 cup cold roast pumpkin
1 handful pecans
1 tsp. cinnamon
1 cup water and ice

- Blend - Enjoy

Lunch and Dinner
Sandwiches

Avocado Reuben Sandwich

2 slices of pumpernickel or whole grain bread
1/2 avocado
1 tsp. organic garlic powder
1 tsp. organic onion powder or 1 Tbsp. grated fresh yellow onion
1 slice of vegan Swiss non-cheese
1/4 cup raw sauerkraut
3 Tbsp. Veganaise grape seed mayo
3 Tbsp. sweet pickle relish
½ cup organic ketchup

- Mix ketchup, relish, garlic powder, onion powder or grated onion and Veganaise mayo in a bowl together. Spread bread with a thin layer of the mixed dressing on both sides of bread.
- Top one side with sauerkraut then place sliced avocado on top of sauerkraut.
- Add non-cheese on other slice of bread.
- Close sandwich. Grill like a grilled cheese sandwich.

Grilled Cheese and Asparagus

2 slices Ezekiel Bread
Vegan margarine
Daiya brand cheddar slices or your favorite non-cheese
2 asparagus spears
Black pepper
Flax Seed

- Pre-heat a sauté pan for the grilled cheese.
- Slab vegan margarine onto the slices of Ezekiel Bread and place a slice of "cheese" on each half. You're cooking two sides at once to conserve Earth's energy.

- Sprinkle with ground flax seed.
- Now add the asparagus, cutting it so it doesn't extend beyond the edges of the sandwich.
- When both sides are brown, glue them together, slice and enjoy with homemade or boxed Pacific brand tomato soup.

Ratatouille Sandwich

1 small eggplant cut in 1-inch pieces
1 small zucchini or yellow summer squash, cut into 3/4-inch slices
1 red pepper cut in strips
1/2 small red onion cut in 1/2-inch wedges
1 Tbsp. EVOO
1/2 tsp. Herbs de Provence or dried thyme, crushed
2 medium plum tomatoes each cut lengthwise in 6 wedges
8 small or 4 large 1/2-inch slices hardy whole wheat or gluten-free, toasted (about 8 oz. total)
1 clove garlic, halved
2 Tbsp. Balsamic vinegar
Fresh thyme sprigs as garnish

- Preheat oven to 400 degrees F. Coat a large shallow roasting pan with nonstick cooking spray. Add eggplant, zucchini, sweet pepper, and onion to prepared pan. Drizzle with olive oil; sprinkle herbs de Provence, 1/8 teaspoon salt, and 1/8 teaspoon black pepper. Toss to coat. Roast vegetables 30 minutes, tossing once.
- Add tomatoes to roasting pan. Roast 15 to 20 minutes more or until vegetables are tender and some surface areas are lightly browned.
- Sprinkle balsamic vinegar over vegetables; toss gently to coat.
- Meanwhile, rub toasted bread with cut sides of the garlic clove. Place two small slices or one large slice of bread one each of the four serving plates.
- Spoon warm vegetable on bread. Garnish with fresh thyme sprigs.

Blissful "Chicken" Salad

8 oz. tempeh
1 cup diced celery
1/2 cup vegan mayo – grape seed works also
2 Tbsp. fresh, not bottled, lemon juice
1/2 tsp. sage
1/8 tsp. oregano
1/2 tsp. rosemary
1/4 tsp. thyme, crushed
1/4 tsp. Himalayan salt to taste

- Steam tempeh 10 minutes. Set aside to cool.
- In a small bowl whisk together remaining ingredients.
- Cut steamed tempeh into 1/4 inch cubes.
- Toss gently with dressing and chill.
- Adjust seasonings if needed and serve on whole grain or gluten-free bread.

Raw Tacos

Taco "meat"
1 cup raw walnuts (preferably soaked & rehydrated)
1 Tbsp. Bragg's Liquid Amino's
1 tsp. EVOO
1 tsp. ground cumin
Dash cayenne pepper

Raw salsa
1 Large, firm vine-ripened tomato, seeds removed and roughly chopped
½ red bell pepper, seeds removed and chopped
½ red onion, diced
¼ cup fresh cilantro, roughly chopped
1 clove garlic, minced
½ lime, juiced
1 Tbsp. EVOO
1 tsp. raw honey
1/8 – 1/4 tsp. salt
½ avocado, chopped
romaine lettuce leaves, washed and pat dry

- To make the taco meat: Place the walnuts into a food processor and pulse a few times. Add the rest of the ingredients and pulse a few more times, just enough so everything is combined but still has texture.
- To make the salsa: Toss all of the ingredients into a large bowl and stir to combine. This is best after it's had time to sit to let the flavors meld (a couple of hours in the fridge would work), but it can also be used immediately.
To assemble the tacos: Tear off large Romaine leaves for the taco shell. Layer the taco with the taco "meat," salsa, and chopped avocado.

Saturday Sloppy Joes

Sloppy sauce:
2 medium onions
1 Tbsp. yellow mustard
1 tsp. Stevia or maple syrup
1 Cup tomato sauce
1 Tbsp. Cider vinegar
1/2 tsp. wheat-free sauce

Joe:
1 Cake of crumbled tempeh
1 cup of cooked, long grain brown rice
Virgin olive oil or expeller-pressed vegetable oil
1 Tbsp. chili powder
1 Stalk of celery, minced
1 Medium onion, minced
1 Pinch of cayenne powder
1 ½ cup of vegetable stock
Wheat-free soy sauce or Tamari

- In a sauté pan, add a tsp. of oil; gently brown the tempeh, breaking it up with the back of a fork.
- In the same sauté pan, add a bit more oil, then gently sauté the onions and celery for 1 minute over medium high heat.
- Now, add the stock to the sauté pan.

- Add the sloppy Joe sauce, cooked rice, cayenne, salt and pepper, and then adjust taste and consistency.
- Serve over whole-wheat buns and tope with creamy cole slaw.

Tempeh "Tuna" Salad
Gluten-free
serves 2-3

1 Package organic tempeh
1/4 cup onions, diced
1/4 cup celery, diced
2 Tbsp. Dill, chopped
1 Tbsp. Veganaise Mayonnaise
2 tsp. Spicy mustard
2 tsp. Lemon juice
1 Pinch cayenne
½ sheet Nori, powdered in a coffee grinder
Sea salt and pepper to taste

- Boil the tempeh in a medium-sized pot for 20 minutes, until tender.
- Drain the water and let tempeh cool.
- Meanwhile, chop the vegetables and dill.
- Once tempeh has cooled smash it with a fork, your hands, or any mashing utensil you have in your kitchen.
- Smash it until it's mostly broken apart.
- Mix in all other ingredients and refrigerate until ready to use.

Mediterranean Portobello Burger
4 servings

Looking for a healthy grilling alternative? This open-faced mushroom sandwich comes topped with a luscious Greek-style salad. A mushroom burger is a far healthier option than the 195 calories a greasy ground beef patty provides. Serve with cucumber spears and a glass of icy-cold white wine.

1 clove garlic, minced (anti-cancer)

½ tsp. Sea salt
2 Tbsp. EVOO, divided
4 Portobello mushroom caps, stems and gills removed
4 gluten-free flat buns
½ cup sliced roasted red peppers
½ cup chopped tomatoes (lycopene)
¼ cup crumbled reduced-fat feta cheese
2 Tbsp. chopped pitted Kalamata olives
1 tsp. red wine vinegar
½ tsp. dried oregano
2 cups loosely packed mixed baby salad-greens

- Preheat grill to medium-high.
- Mash garlic and salt on a cutting board with side of knife until it's a smooth paste. Mix the paste with 1 tablespoon oil in a small bowl.
- Lightly brush the oil mixture over the Portabella mushrooms and on one side of each slice of bread.
- Combine red peppers, tomatoes, feta, olives, vinegar, oregano and remaining 1 tablespoon oil in a medium bowl.
- Grill or sauté the mushroom caps until tender, about 4 minutes per side. Grill the bread until crisp, about 1 minute per side.
- Toss salad greens with the red pepper mixture.
- Place the grilled mushrooms top-side down on 4 half-slices of the flat bread. Top with the salad mixture and the remaining bread.
- Boom!

"Sprouting" Sunshine Pita Pocket
Serves 4

Sprouts have long been famous as healthy food but recent research shows in addition to being a wonderful source of nutrients, they also have a groovy curative ability. Sprouts, like alfalfa, radish, broccoli, and clover contain intense amounts of phytochemicals (plant compounds) that can protect us against disease. Sprouts also contain a constellation of highly active antioxidants that prevent DNA destruction and protect us from the ongoing effects of aging.

1 head of cauliflower, processed into powder
1/4 tsp. dry mustard
1/2 lemon, juiced
1/2 tsp. curry powder
1/2 tsp. powdered kelp
1/4 tsp. ground cardamom
1/3 cup Veganaise mayonnaise or substitute
4 ounces alfalfa sprouts
3 carrots, grated
2 tomatoes, sliced
2 large gluten-free pita breads

- In a food processer pulse the washed and drained cauliflower into dust; add listed ingredients through mayonnaise and mix.
- Chill well. Spread mix in pita bread and add your favorite sprouts, carrots and tomatoes.

Abundant ways to serve sprouts
- Add to tossed salads
- Use in coleslaw (cabbage, clover, radish)
- Try in potato salad (mung bean, lentil)
- Try in wraps and roll-ups (alfalfa, sunflower, radish)
- Stir-fry with other vegetables (alfalfa, clover, radish, mung bean, lentil)
- Blend into fruit shakes or juices (cabbage, mung bean, lentil)
- Blend with vegetable juices (cabbage, mung bean, lentil)
- Replace celery in sandwich spreads (lentil, radish)
- Mix with soft cheeses for a dip (mung bean, radish)
- Grind up and use in sandwich spreads (lentil, radish)
- Top grilled cheese sandwiches after grilling (alfalfa, clover)
- Stir into soups or stews when serving (mung bean, lentil)

- Mix into pancake or waffle batter (buckwheat)
- Eat them fresh and uncooked in a sprout salad (salad mixes)
- Top omelet or scrambled eggs (alfalfa, clover, radish)
- Combine in rice dishes (fenugreek, lentil, mung bean)
- Add to sushi (radish, sunflower)
- Sauté with onions (mung bean, clover, radish)
- Puree with peas or beans (mung bean, lentil)
- Add to baked beans (lentil)
- Steam and serve with butter (mung bean, lentil)
- Use in sandwiches instead of Iceberg lettuce (alfalfa, clover, radish)

Grilled Vegetable Sandwich
4 servings

¼ cup light Veganaise or Hain brand expeller pressed mayonnaise
2 Tbsp. chopped fresh basil
2 Tbsp. garlic, chopped
2 tsp. fresh lemon juice
1 medium red onion, cut into 4 slices
1 large red bell pepper, cut into 8 slices
1 large zucchini, cut on an angle into 8 slices
2 tsp. EVOO
¼ tsp. sea salt
¼ tsp. freshly ground pepper
8 slices Ezekiel or Udi's gluten-free bread
¾ cup hummus
1 medium organic tomato, cut into 8 slices

- In a small bowl, combine the mayonnaise, basil, garlic, and lemon juice. Set aside.

- Coat the grill rack with cooking spray. Preheat the grill. Brush the onion, bell pepper and zucchini with the olive oil. Sprinkle with salt and pepper.
- Place the onion and peppers on the rack and grill for 10 to 12 minutes, turning once, or until the vegetables are well marked and tender. Place the zucchini slices on the rack and cook for 6 to 8 minutes, turning once, or until marked and tender.
- Equally spread 4 slices of the bread with the hummus and place on a cutting board. Top each with an onion slice separated into rings, 2 bell pepper slices, 2 zucchini slices and 2 tomato slices. Spread the remaining bread slices with the mayonnaise mixture and place on top of the tomatoes.

Vegetables can be grilled the day before, wrapped tightly and stored in the refrigerator until ready to use.

Chipotle Black Bean Burgers
Yield: 6 servings (serving size: 1 burger)

1 (15-ounce) Can black beans, rinsed and drained
1 cup mashed cooked sweet potatoes (about 1 large sweet potato, peeled)
¼ cup oat flour (see recipe note)
½ Tbsp. dried parsley
¼ tsp. chipotle chili pepper seasoning
¼ tsp. garlic powder
¼ tsp. sea salt
1/8 tsp. pepper

- Preheat oven to broil setting.
- With a potato masher or fork, mash black beans in a large bowl, leaving about ¼ of the beans whole. Mix in sweet potatoes, oat flour, parsley, chipotle chile pepper seasoning, garlic powder, salt, and pepper.
- Scoop out 1/3 cup of bean mixture, and place on an 11 x 17-inch baking sheet that has been rubbed with olive

oil. Flatten and shape into a circle with spatula. Repeat with the remaining bean mixture to make 6 burgers.

- Broil 4 inches from heat about 7-8 minutes or until golden brown. Flip burgers carefully with spatula. Broil 2-3 more minutes, and serve.

Zesty Dragon Bowl

1 zucchini, cubed
1 cup shredded carrots
1 cup chopped broccoli
Sea salt and black pepper to taste
3 Tbsp. virgin coconut oil
½ cup dried fruit, chopped
½ cup sun-dried tomatoes, chopped
1 Jalapeno pepper, minced
Slivered almonds for garnish
Green onions, chopped for garnish
¼ cup slivered basil leaves
4 cups fresh arugula
2 Tbsp. unsweetened coconut flakes

- Prep all the veggies, dried fruit, jalapeno and sun-dried tomatoes.
- Heat the coconut oil over medium heat and add the vegetables, nuts, and dried fruit.
- Stir-fry very briefly - no more than 1 minute, stirring constantly. Do not let veggies get soft and mushy. You want crispiness.
- Add 1 cup cooked brown rice, season with salt and pepper.
- Dispense equally into 2 to 3 bowls lined with arugula leaves; garnish with almonds, basil, coconut flakes and green onions.
- Bon appetite!

Soups

Red Lentil Soup with Curry and Coconut
4 to 6 servings

Red lentils cook very rapidly, so don't walk away from the pot for too long. Protein-rich lentils digest quite easily and compliment digestion. Curry contains turmeric, a powerful anti-inflammatory and liver cleanser. In India, where folks eat it daily, Alzheimer's disease is hardly known.

3 Tbsp. raw, un-refined coconut oil
3 medium onions, coarsely chopped
1 cup red lentils, washed and rinsed
3 medium carrots; roughly chopped
14 oz. can coconut milk
1 bay leaf
3 garlic cloves, minced
1 inch piece of fresh ginger, grated
1 Tbsp. curry powder
½ cup chopped cilantro

- In a medium non-corrosive saucepan, over low fire, heat the coconut oil. Add the onions, cook, and stir for 1 minute.
- Add 4 cups filtered water, lentils, carrots, coconut milk, salt and bay leaf. Cover and bring to a low simmer stirring often, about 15 minutes.
- Meanwhile, back at the ranch, heat the remaining 1 Tbsp. oil over low heat. Add garlic, ginger and curry. Gently cook for 2 minutes, stirring frequently. Add to soup.
- Remove bay leaf. In a food processor, blender, or with an electric whisk, puree in batches until velvety smooth. Taste and adjust salt.
- Garnish with chopped fresh cilantro and serve with pride.

Chilled Corn Bisque with Curry Oil

On a hot day you don't want to turn on the stove. Instead, prepare this refreshing chilled corn soup. Keep yourself and the kitchen cool as a lake breeze with this simple-to-prepare, refreshing, cold soup.

Early settlers may have perished if the Native Americans hadn't turned them on to corn. Settlers learned to grow it by planting kernels in small holes fertilized with small fish. Wise Native Americans celebrated corn's health mojo.

3 cups sweet corn kernels
1 cup almond or coconut milk
Sea salt or Himalayan Salt

Garnish
½ cup sweet corn kernels
Julienne zucchini

Curry Infused Olive Oil
Warm, but do not boil ¾ cups olive oil in saucepan

Add 3 Tbsp. of curry or to taste.
Whisk well and shut off heat.
Let set overnight then strain through cheese cloth or fine mesh strainer.

Bisque:
- In high-speed blender or food processor, combine the corn, salt and almond milk, puree until smooth.
- Pass through a fine mesh sieve and season to taste with salt and pepper.
- If you wish, do not strain and leave in the fibrous pulp. It's not going to kill you.
- Portion then garnish with julienne zucchini and kernels of corn. Drizzle with curry-infused olive oil.

Winter Vegetable Stew

Serve this economical, robust stew with gluten-free or an authentic rye bread and a dark green bitter greens salad for the perfect balance of wholesome, healing winter nutrition.

1 leek, washed and trimmed
1 medium onion
1 Tbsp. extra virgin olive, grape seed, or walnut oil
2 carrots, unpeeled
½ tsp. nutmeg
½ jalapeno pepper, chopped
½ tsp. cinnamon
2 cups diced butternut squash
2 Yukon Gold potatoes, washed
1 oven roasted sweet potato
1/4 Cup chopped cilantro and parsley
1 box vegetable stock

- Cut all veggies approximately the same size: bite size.
- Chop the herbs and reserve.
- Briefly, over medium-high heat, sauté the veggies, spices, and jalapeno, in a scant amount of olive oil. DO NOT OVER-COOK the veggies; leave them a bit firm.
- Pour in the stock and bring to a simmer, then shut off the heat.
- Serve in warmed soup bowl and garnish with a tablespoon of chopped herbs.
- Tastes great the second day, too.

Green Chili Tortilla Soup

2 large zucchini, chopped coarsely
1 Anaheim green chili, chopped coarsely
1/2 pound green chili, diced
2 Tbsp. minced garlic
1/2 cup chopped cilantro
4 corn tortillas (Non-GMO)

1/2 cup loosely packed oregano leaves
1 Tbsp. vegetable broth seasoning
1 lime, quartered

- Place everything, except the cilantro, corn tortillas, and oregano leaves, into a large pot and cover with filtered water.
- Bring it to a boil and simmer for 5 minutes.
- Add sea salt or Bragg's Liquid Amino to taste at the last minute.
- Serve garnished with chopped cilantro, oregano leaves, and a squeeze of fresh lime.

Vegan Mushroom Soup

2 Tbsp. EVOO
8 oz. fresh, stemmed shiitake or mini Bella mushrooms, washed and sliced
1 Small onion, chopped
Sea salt and pepper to taste
2 cloves of garlic, minced
2 cups almond or coconut milk (reserve 1/4 cup)
1 heaping Tbsp. potato starch

- In a 2 quart pan sauté the mushrooms, onions, garlic, salt and pepper in olive oil.
- Add all but 1/4 cup of almond or cashew milk into a mixing bowl. Mix in potato starch and let dissolve into a slurry.
- Add to the mushroom mixture mushroom mix and cook over medium-low heat, stirring often until thickened.
- Make it a day ahead for a tasty green bean casserole ingredient.

Lima Bean Soup
Serves 4

3 cups cooked lima beans
3 cups vegetable stock
2 Tbsp. EVOO
1 large onion, chopped
1 cup carrots, chopped
1 Tbsp. garbanzo bean flour

1 tsp. sea salt or Himalayan salt
1 tsp. dried thyme or 2 Tbsp. fresh thyme leaves
1 cup plain almond or coconut milk

- Puree beans with liquid until smooth and set aside
- In a large soup pot, heat the oil and sauté onion, carrot, over medium-low heat for 5 minutes
- Stir in the flour and salt, then pour in the almond milk and whisk constantly until mixture thickens
- Reduced heat to low and stir in the pureed beans.
- Garnish with fresh thyme leaves then serve with a dark leafy green salad

Salads, Vegetables, Sides, and Fruits

Spinach Salad with Beets and Oranges
The kids will dig it!

2 Navel oranges, peeled
6 cups torn spinach, washed
3 cups shredded peeled beets (about 1 pound)
3 Tbsp. minced shallot
1/4 cup raspberry vinegar
1/4 tsp. freshly ground black pepper
1/4 cup minced fresh chives

- Peel oranges, and cut each crosswise into 5 slices. Place spinach on a large platter.
- Spoon beets onto spinach, and arrange orange slices on beets.
- In a small bowl, stir together the raspberry vinegar, shallots and pepper. Drizzle over salad.
- Garnish the attractive salad with chives.
- Serve with pride.

Polynesian Coconut Bowl Salad

1 cup fresh ripe organic pineapple, cut into small chunks
3/4 cup fresh organic ruby red grapefruit, cut into small chunks
1 large ripe organic kiwi, peel and cut into medium chunks

1 organic orange, peel and cut into medium chunks
1 ripe organic banana, peel and slice into medium size rounds
1 small ripe organic avocado, cut into medium chunks
1/2 ripe organic lemon
1/4 cup fresh organic coconut meat shreds
2 empty and clean coconut shell halves

- In a large bowl, mix together your pineapple, grapefruit, kiwi, orange and banana chunks.
- In a different bowl add your avocado chunks. With a vegetable peeler, remove the zest from the Meyer lemon into long strips.
- Zest the lemon and reserve. Squeeze the lemon juice on to the avocado chunks and gently stir to completely coat.
- Do not mash
- Add the coated avocado to the other fruit and gently mix well, creating your fruit mix.
- In each coconut half place 1/2 of the fruit mix in. It may overfill
- Garnish with the coconut shreds and lemon zest

Broccoli and Tempeh "Anti-Cancer" Salad with Peanut Dressing

2 cups washed greens of choice. A blend of wild greens is best
1 cup each washed chopped broccoli and cauliflower florets, snap peas, diced pepper
1 unpeeled, grated carrot
1 red bell pepper
Sunflower seeds
½ cup raisins
Green onion, chopped
Tempeh – cubed – lightly sautéed in olive oil, honey and ginger to coat

Dressing:
2-3 Tbsp. organic peanut butter
1 tsp. minced, peeled, ginger (use a food grater)
1 ½ tsp. fresh lemon juice
Water as needed for consistency

Puree in blender
Add salt and pepper to taste

- Cut tempeh into ½ inch cubes
- In a skillet, warm the tempeh cubes in olive oil, honey and fresh ginger. Not too long.
- Toss tempeh plus remaining ingredients into a large salad bowl and toss with the dressing.

Crispy Crunchy Summer Salad

1/2 head red cabbage, shredded
1/2 head white cabbage, shredded
1/2 cup sliced almonds
2 Tbsp. sesame seeds

Dressing:
1/3 cup tamari (wheat free for gluten sensitive folks)
2 Tbsp. rice wine vinegar
1 Tbsp. toasted sesame oil
2 Tbsp. EVOO
2 Tbsp. maple syrup
1/2 Lemon
Sea salt or Himalayan salt and pepper to taste

- In a small mixing bowl, combine tamari, rice wine vinegar, maple syrup, and whisk in the sesame oil. Set aside.
- Shred cabbage into thin strips in a large mixing bowl.
- Toast almonds and sesame seeds in a small pan. Toss toasted sesame seeds and sliced almonds into the cabbage bowl.
- Add the tamari/maple dressing, salt and pepper. Squeeze in ½ of the lemon and stir together. Store in the fridge to cool, approximately one hour.

Quinoa Walnut Cherry Salad
6 servings

Nuts to you! If you take a gander at a shelled walnut, you'll notice it looks appropriately like your brain. Walnuts have often been thought of as a "brain food," not only because of the wrinkled brain-like appearance of their meat and shells, but because of their dense concentration of Omega-3 essential fatty acids. Our brains are more than 60% structural fat. For your gray matter to function properly, fat needs to be primarily the Omega-3 fats found in walnuts, flaxseed and cold-water fish.

4 cups of cooked quinoa
1/3 cup olive oil
1/2 cup chopped red onion
1 red pepper, diced
1/2 cup dried cherries or fresh in season
¼ cup fresh lemon juice
1/4 cup fresh chopped mint
Himalayan salt and cracked black pepper to taste
1/2 cup toasted walnuts, chopped
Several leafs of butter lettuce for a bed

- Cook and drain the quinoa of liquid, then add quinoa to a mixing bowl.
- Add the remaining ingredients and fluff with fork.
- Place the lettuce around the edge of a serving bowl or platter, then mound the salad in the center and serve.

Asian Quinoa with Summer Vegetables

Use a variety of in-season vegetables. Nuts and dried fruit give this a crunchy, sweet and savory flavor.

1 cup quinoa, rinsed
2 cups water
1 cup green beans, Slices
1/2 cup broccoli florets
1/2 cup cauliflower florets
1/2 onion, chopped
1 Tbsp. EVOO
1 tsp. ground ginger or ½ inch fresh

1 garlic clove, minced
1/2 tsp. sea salt or Himalayan salt
1 Tbsp. wheat-free soy sauce
Hot pepper flakes

- Rinse quinoa and place in saucepan with 2 cups water. Bring to boil and then reduce heat to medium for 18 minutes stirring every few minutes. Add soy sauce and stir once all water has been absorbed.
- In sauté pan cook onion, broccoli, cauliflower in EVOO until softened 1-2 minutes. Add ginger. This would be when you add the hot pepper flakes.
- Add 2 dashes of soy sauce to vegetables and stir mixture together. Serve on top of finished soy-flavored Quinoa or mix it up together.
- This recipe would be perfect topped with some grilled and diced tempeh, as well. Walnuts on top would be outstanding.
- Enjoy! Serves 3-4 large servings of protein-packed deliciousness!

Mediterranean Quinoa Salad

3 cups cooked quinoa
1/2 cup Greek black olives, pitted
1 Tbsp. ground flax seed
2 cloves garlic, crushed
1/2 cup chopped scallions
1 cup cherry tomatoes, halved
1 cup cucumber, chopped
1/2 cup radish, chopped
2 Tbsp. fresh mint
2 Tbsp. cilantro, chopped
1 cup chopped parsley
1 Small bunch watercress, chopped
1/4 cup freshly squeezed lemon juice
1/4 cup extra virgin olive oil
1/2 cup crumbled feta or goats cheese
Himalayan salt and pepper to taste

- Cook, drain and allow quinoa cool to room temperature, then transfer to a serving bowl.

- Mix the garlic and scallions thoroughly with the quinoa and add the remaining chopped herbs and vegetables. Stir in the lemon juice and extra virgin olive oil.
- Finally, mix in the feta cheese and olives then season with freshly ground salt and pepper.
- Set aside for at least 30 minutes before serving to allow the flavors to gently blend.

Jicama-Orange Salad with Summer Berries
Low-Glycemic—Appropriate for Diabetics
Serves 8

We already know the romantic magic of eating berries warm off the vine. The anthocyanins, which give them their deep color, are the heroes' that are brimming with phytochemicals, especially, antioxidants which protect us from cancer, age related eye disorders, and a constellation of degenerative diseases. Blueberries, loaded with vitamin C, manganese, fiber, and vitamin E. Berries can be tossed into granola, smoothies, yogurt, stir-fry's, but not with snarky Cool Whip. Wash them first then eat them like candy. They also protect against colon and ovarian cancer.

1/3 cup fresh lime juice
1 tsp. sea salt or Himalayan salt
1 tsp. Chili powder
Cayenne pepper to taste
1 pound of jicama, the Mexican potato, peeled and diced
Mandarin oranges, drained
2 minced green onions
Blue and red raspberries for garnish

- In a large bowl, mix the lime, salt, Chile powder and cayenne together.
- Add the peeled and diced Jicama, oranges, green onions and toss to coat.
- Place into a pretty glass bowl, and top with berries.
- Serve chilled. Do not attempt to mix the berries into the salad. They will break down and ruin the looks of the colorful dish.

Health benefits of Jicama - Asthma: Vitamin C, antioxidant and anti-inflammatory - A large study has shown that young children with asthma experience significantly less wheezing if they eat a diet high in fruits rich in vitamin C.

Hoosier Summer Tomato, Basil, and Corn Vegetable Salad

Want something to do with all those tomatoes, corn, and basil exploding off the vine? This season improve your family's health while supporting the local economy by purchasing tomatoes and corn locally. The longer vegetables are on the vine, the more sun-drenched nutrition they contain. Why would we eat vegetables that were picked three weeks ago, shipped 2,000 miles and then ripened by way of un-natural gassing methods that only increase color, not nutrition? I didn't think so.

1 Stalk celery, washed and coarsely chopped
1 Bunch of green onions, washed and chopped
2 Large fresh vine ripe tomatoes cut into eights
1 Bunch of basil cut into strips
1 cup pinto beans, drained
1 cup of fresh non-GMO corn sliced off the cob. (Does not need to be cooked)
3 Tbsp. Red wine vinegar
1 Tbsp. Ground flax seed
½ cup EVOO
Himalayan salt and pepper to taste

- Gently mix all ingredients together in a large bowl and refrigerate until you serve this colorful taste of summer.

Avocado on the Half-Shell – The Alligator Pear

1 ripe avocado
1 Tbsp. balsamic vinegar
3 cloves of chopped raw garlic
Himalayan salt and black pepper

- Mix balsamic, garlic, salt and pepper.
- Halve the avocado and remove the stone.
- Cupping ½ of the avocado in your palm cut the avocado into cubes with a paring knife, leaving the

avocado meat in the shell. Try not to penetrate the alligator shell with the knife.
- Pour mixture over cubed avocado and eat right out of the shell

Spicy Thai Style Slaw
Makes 4 servings

2 cups thinly shredded cabbage (Napa Cabbage works too)
1 cup bean sprouts
1 large carrot (julienned)
1 red, green, or yellow pepper (thinly sliced)
2 green onions (sliced)
1 handful cilantro (chopped)
1 handful mint (chopped)
Use a variety of the vegetables you prefer

Dressing:
1 Tbsp. coconut milk
¼ Cup organic peanut butter
1 Tbsp. wheat-free soy sauce
1 juice from one lime
1 Tbsp. toasted sesame oil
1 Tbsp. Stevia powder or 2 Tbsp. raw honey
1 hot chili, finely chopped
1 Tbsp. roasted peanuts, chopped

- Mix the cabbage, bean sprouts, carrot, peppers, green onion, cilantro and mint in a large bowl.
- Mix the coconut milk, fish sauce, peanut butter, toasted sesame oil, lime juice, Stevia and chili in a small mixing bowl.
- Toss the salad with the dressing and sprinkle with chopped peanuts.

Sweet and Sour Kale Salad

This kale salad holds up a lot longer than lettuce once it's dressed, so if you end up getting a late start on dinner your salad won't get soggy.

1 bunch kale
2 nectarines or peaches
¼ lb. dried cherries or cranberries
¼ lb. pine nuts
¼ cup EVOO
¼ cup Bragg's apple cider vinegar
Himalayan salt and pepper to taste

- Chop the kale as finely as possible; it's worth the effort.
- Cut nectarines or peaches into small chunks and add them to the kale.
- Add pine nuts and dried cherries or cranberries.
- Add olive oil, vinegar, sea salt and pepper.
- Toss and serve.

<u>Sicilian Garden Salad</u>
Serves 4

2 large, ripe organic tomatoes cut into eights
1 small Bermuda onion cut into half-circles
Pinch of sea salt and coarse black pepper
2 Tbsp. ground flax seeds
2 cucumbers, sliced
1 cup of julienne spinach leaves
1/2 cup slivered almonds
1/4 cup of freshly chopped basil
1 Tbsp. fresh oregano leaves
Several splashes of red wine or balsamic vinegar
2 Tbsp. EVOO

- Wash the produce as if your family's lives depended on it.
- Place the sun-drenched vegetables into a lovely salad bowl.
- Add the fresh herbs, then drizzle with the extra virgin olive oil and vinegar and gently toss.
- Give the flavors time to consummate their marriage.
- Serve either cold or at room temperature.

Kale and Grapefruit Salad

1 bunch of kale washed and de-stemmed
2 pink grapefruits, juiced
2 Tbsp. chia seeds

Dressing:
1 lemon, juiced
1/3 cup grape seed oil or your favorite Expeller-pressed oil
1 tsp. Himalayan salt
1/4 tsp. cayenne pepper
2 tsp. maple syrup

- Place kale in a large bowl.
- Mix the remaining ingredients in a medium bowl until well incorporated.
- Mix dressing ingredients - pour dressing over the kale and serve.

Spicy Orange Slaw

2 cups grated carrots (do not peel)
2 cups shredded purple cabbage
1/2 cup chopped cilantro
1/4 cup roasted pumpkin seeds
3 Tbsp. fresh orange juice
1 Tbsp. fresh lime juice
1/2 tsp. ground cumin
1/4 tsp. cayenne pepper
1/4 tsp. Himalayan salt

- Combine all ingredients in a medium bowl and mix thoroughly.

Dairy-Free Ranch Dressing via My Whole Food Life

1 cup cashews (raw and unsalted)
1/4 cup almond or oat milk (If you like a super thick dressing, just omit the milk)
1 clove garlic minced
3 Tbsp. chives finely chopped
3 Tbsp. Parsley finely chopped

3 tsp. white wine vinegar
Himalayan salt to taste

- Add ingredients to food processor and blend until desired thickness. Pour over your favorite salad and enjoy!

Sweet Curry Dressing with Tahini

2 Tbsp. tahini
½ tsp. curry powder
2 Tbsp. maple syrup/honey
1 Tbsp. EVOO
½ Tbsp. fresh lime juice
4 Tbsp. water

- Mix all the ingredients together in a food processor or blender to make a thick creamy dressing. Serve over your favorite salad. Dressing will keep refrigerated up to one week in an airtight bottle.

Coconut Mayonnaise
Makes 1 1/2 cups
For sandwiches, dips, salads and spreads

1 whole, local egg
2 local egg yolks
1 Tbsp. mustard
1 Tbsp. fresh lemon juice
½ tsp. Himalayan salt
¼ tsp. pepper
½ cup EVOO
½ cup virgin coconut oil (melted, if solid)

- Place whole egg plus 2 egg yolks, mustard, lemon juice, salt, and pepper into a food processor or blender. Blend briefly for a few seconds.
- With the processor or blender running on low speed, start adding your oils very slowly. Start out with drops and then work up to a steady light stream. This will take a few minutes.

- Continue blending until all the oil is used up and there is no free standing oil.

Vodka Spiked Cherry Tomatoes with Pepper Salt

Remember: Too much broth spoils the cook! This is a great side dish.

2 pints cherry or grape tomatoes stemmed, cut in half
¼ cup vodka
½ cup chopped herbs
2 Tbsp. White-wine or rice vinegar
1 Tbsp. raw honey, Stevia, or xylitol
1 tsp. grated lemon peel zest
3 Tbsp. Himalayan salt
1 Tbsp. cracked black pepper

- Stir the vodka, sweetener, herbs, white-wine vinegar and zest together in a mixing bowl. Pour in the tomatoes and gently mix.
- Marinate for 30 minutes to an hour, garnish with salt and pepper and serve them as an appetizer to a summer supper with great friends.

Tomato Quinoa Risotto
Serves 6

1 cup washed and rinsed quinoa seed
1 cup tomato sauce
1 cup water or vegetable stock
½ medium onion, diced
5 garlic cloves, minced
1-1/2 cups diced fresh Roma tomatoes
15 ounces cannelloni beans
2 Tbsp. EVOO
Himalayan salt and pepper to taste
Fresh slivered basil as garnish

- In a medium pot, bring the tomato sauce and water or vegetable stock to a boil and add quinoa. Reduce heat

to a medium-low simmer. Add the onion and garlic and sauté for 2 minutes.
- Continue cooking until all the liquid is absorbed. (about 15-20 minutes).
- Stir in drained beans, tomatoes, EVOO, sea salt and pepper and let sit about 2 minutes to soften the tomatoes. Garnish with basil and serve.

Vegan Tempeh Potato Patties
Makes 6 patties

4 ounces tempeh (about 1/2 cup)
1 cup vegetable stock
1/4 - 1/2 cup onion, chopped
1 Tbsp. garlic, minced
Himalayan salt and pepper to taste
2 Tbsp. non-dairy butter spread
1 cup mashed potatoes

- In a small saucepan, add tempeh to vegetable stock. Cook for 10 minutes. Remove tempeh and cool slightly.
- Heat butter in a large skillet. Add onion and cook over medium heat for 2-3 minutes.
- In the meantime, add mashed potatoes to a large bowl. Crumble tempeh into potatoes. Flavor as desired with a few squirts of Bragg Liquid Aminos, garlic, salt and pepper. Combine well. Form into patties and add to hot pan.
- Brown patties on each side over medium high heat, turning only once carefully.

Tangy Marinated Vegetables

Marinade:
1/2 cup expeller-pressed vegetable oil
1/4 cup extra virgin olive oil
2 cloves of freshly chopped garlic
1/4 cup red wine or rice vinegar
2 Tbsp. dried oregano or ¼ cup fresh oregano leaves
2 Tbsp. dried or ¼ cup fresh basil
2 Tbsp. fresh chopped parsley
1/2 tsp. dried cayenne pepper flakes

Vegetables:
2 cups broccoli florets
1 cup diced carrots, unpeeled
1 cup of button mushrooms, cut into quarters
1 cup frozen peas
1 red bell pepper, 1/4 inch dice
1 cup lima beans
1/2 red onion, diced

- Pour marinade into a 2-quart canning jar with lid. Tupperware works, too.
- Refrigerate 4 hours or overnight, shaking the mixture occasionally.
- Pour over vegetables or enjoy straight from the jar.
- Use these to replace a salty pickle with your next sandwich

Green Beans, Potatoes and Spinach in Coconut Curry

1/3 cup unrefined coconut oil
2 1/2 cups pureed tomatoes
1 1/2 tsp. Himalayan salt
1 tsp. turmeric
1 Tbsp. ground black mustard seeds
1 Tbsp. crushed cayenne pepper (this amount will make it quite spicy, so cut back if you don't want your curry very hot)
1 cup water
1 lb. potatoes, unpeeled, and cut into 1/2 inch cubes
1/2 lb. green beans, trimmed and cut in 1 inch pieces
1/2 cups full-fat coconut milk
1/2 lb. fresh spinach, washed, stemmed, and chopped

- Place oil and tomatoes in a medium pot on medium-high heat and cook for 1 minute. Add salt, turmeric, mustard seeds and cayenne, stir and sauté for 3 to 4 minutes or until the oil glistens in the bubbles of the boiling tomatoes.
- Stir in water and potatoes and bring to a boil. Reduce the heat to low, cover and cook for 10 minutes.
- Remove the lid and stir in the green beans. Cover and cook an additional 5 to 8 minutes or until potatoes are cooked through.

- Stir in coconut milk and increase heat to medium. Bring to a boil, then stir in spinach, cover and reduce the heat to low. Cook for 1 minute, or until spinach wilts into the curry. Serve immediately

Seared Green Beans with Garlic and Chiles

2 Tbsp. expeller-pressed peanut oil
1 Lb. trimmed and washed green beans
3 cloves of minced garlic
1/4 tsp. hot chili flakes
1 Tbsp. toasted sesame seeds

- Heat a large, deep skillet or wok 2 minutes over medium high heat
- Add oil and swirl to coat the pan
- Increase the heat to high, wait 30 seconds then add the green beans, pepper flakes and a pinch of salt
- Sauté for 3 minutes shaking the pan to move the beans so they cook quickly and evenly
- Stir in garlic, shut off the heat and serve
- Garnish with toasted sesame seeds.

Yellow Basmati Rice

¾ tsp. powdered turmeric
¼ tsp. ground cumin
1 pinch cinnamon
3 cups water
½ tsp. Himalayan salt
2 Tbsp. EVOO
1 ½ cups basmati rice (long grain)
2 Tbsp. chopped scallions for garnish

- In a medium saucepan, heat the turmeric, cumin, and cinnamon over low heat until fragrant, stirring about 30 seconds.
- Add the water, salt, and extra virgin olive oil and bring to a boil. Add the rice and stir well. Cover and reduce heat to a bare simmer.

- Cook covered, without stirring, until the water is absorbed and the rice is tender. (About 20 minutes).
- Remove from the heat and let sit, covered, without stirring, for 10 minutes. Fluff with a fork, add scallions, and serve.

Cilantro-Lime Rice
An easy and delicious rice recipe

If you're a fan of the Chipotle chain, you'll love this! I am always looking for easy recipes - so easy they hardly even qualify as an official "recipe." This is one of the best that even non-cooks can master on the first try. It has three main ingredients - all of which I love! I could literally eat several servings of this rice without an entree.

Long-grain, organic basmati rice
Himalayan salt
Water
Fresh cilantro, stems and all
Fresh limes

- Following directions for the rice you choose and add to your pan. Measure out the water needed for cooking and set aside.
- Wash and cut the stems off the fresh cilantro. I use the same amount of cilantro as I do for rice in a recipe.
- Add the water and cilantro in a blender. On high speed, blend until you have a lovely green cilantro liquid.
- Add the cilantro liquid and rice to your pan. Bring to a boil and then reduce heat and cover. Cook 15 minutes and let stand 5 minutes.
- Squeeze fresh lime juice over the cilantro rice.

Vegetables, Italian Style

Diabetics rejoice! Now is the perfect time to refresh your diet and shrink the waistline simultaneously. Because you have educated yourself, you've learned by now that they're two magic bullets; food and exercise. Did you know the same greasy foods that cause heart disease, also cause Type II diabetes? You'll lose weight, feel more energetic, and keep your glucose readings under control with nature's fresh apothecary. Congratulations. You're on your journey to losing weight and controlling diabetes. Good for you!!

2 small zucchini, cut into 1/2 inch pieces
1 cup organic chopped fresh or canned tomatoes
1/2 pound fresh spring asparagus - snapped into pieces
1/2 small organic cabbage - sliced thin or shredded
2 cups diced red and green peppers, or what every floats your boat
Fresh snow peas, trimmed
1 medium sliced organic onion
1 minced garlic clove
2 Tbsp. EVOO
1 Tbsp. Fresh oregano leaves, chopped fine
1 Tbsp. Fresh rosemary leaves, chopped fine
Juice of I lime

- Wash and trim vegetables. Slice zucchini into 1/2 inch pieces, snap asparagus into pieces, thinly slice, or shred cabbage. Red cabbage is cool, but it will make everything purple.
- Heat the olive oil in frying pan and slowly cook the onion over medium heat until soft. Add vegetables, lime juice, rosemary and oregano.
- Cook over medium heat for 3 minutes, keeping some crunch to the vegetables. Add chopped tomatoes at the last minute of cooking. Stir occasionally.
- Serve immediately.

Zucchini and Potato Hash Browns

1 pound red potatoes, grated
1 medium yellow squash, grated
1 Medium zucchini, grated
1 Small onion, finely chopped
4 Cloves garlic, minced
1 tsp. Himalayan salt

1/4 tsp. pepper
1 Tbsp. EVOO

- If you have a food processor, run the potatoes, yellow squash, zucchini, onion, and garlic through it on the grate setting. If you don't have a food processor, you can use a box grater to grate the vegetables.
- Squeeze the excess moisture from the vegetables. (Removing the liquid is essential to making crispy hash browns).
- Add the seasoned salt and pepper to the vegetables and stir to thoroughly combine.
- Add oil to a largest skillet you have. Spread the hash brown mixture evenly over the bottom of the pan. Cook over a medium high flame until the bottom is crispy, approximately 4 – 6 minutes. Then flip and cook until the other side is crispy, approximately 4 – 6 minutes.

Notes:
*If you have a waffle iron, you can try cooking the grated vegetables in it. Brush or spray with oil.

*Place 1/2 cup of grated veggies over each square on the waffle maker. Spread evenly over the bottom of the waffle maker, lock the lid down, and cook for 8 – 10 minutes or until the hash browns are crispy and cooked through.

Cranberry Salsa

1 (12 ounce) bag cranberries, fresh or frozen
1 bunch cilantro, chopped
1 bunch green onions cut into 3 inch lengths
1 jalapeno pepper, seeded and minced
2 limes, juiced
3/4 cup Sucanat, Stevia powder
1 pinch salt

- Wash the cranberries, green onions, pepper and lime to remove field contaminants.
- Combine cranberries, cilantro, green onions, jalapeno

pepper,
lime juice, sugar, and salt in the bowl of a food processor.
Chop or pulse to medium consistency. Don't turn it into a
soup. Cover and refrigerate if not using immediately.

- Serve at room temperature as you would regular salsa or
  spread it on that dried out holiday fruit cake.
- Use as a topping for a tempeh steak or as a hors d'oeurve
  or crostini topping.

Pico De Gallo

6 medium non-GMO Farmer's Market tomatoes, diced
1 medium yellow onion, diced
1/4 cup cilantro chopped
Juice of (1) lime
2 fresh serrano or jalapeño seeded and minced
1 tsp. minced fresh garlic
Himalayan salt to taste

- Put all ingredients in a bowl and mix well. Let set a few
  minutes.

Mini Zucchini "Cheese" Bites

2 cups grated zucchini (about 1 medium)
1 local fresh egg
½ cup nutritional yeast flakes
¼ cup chopped cilantro
Himalayan salt and black pepper to taste

- Preheat oven to 400 degrees.
- Spray a mini muffin pan with nonstick cooking spray. In
  a bowl mix the zucchini, egg, cheese and cilantro. You
  do not have to add any salt or pepper since the
  Parmesan is salty enough.
- Evenly divide the mixture into the mini muffin pan filling
  to the top, packed down in each cup.
- Bake for 15- 18 minutes until golden brown around the
  edges.

Raw Avocado Bites

1 avocado (pitted and diced)
1/3 Cup nutritional yeast flakes
1 Tbsp. smoked paprika
1 tsp. garlic powder

- Mix last 3 ingredients then toss with avocado until evenly coated!

Cauliflower Tortillas / Soft Taco Wraps

1 head of washed cauliflower
4 local eggs
1/2 tsp. Himalayan alt
3/4 tsp. garlic granules
1/2 tsp. Mexican seasoning/spices (optional)

- Cut the cauliflower into florets
- Add 1/2 of the florets to a food processor and pulse until they are a crumb-like texture, then pulse a little further until a fine texture is achieved. Remove the cauliflower and add it to a steamer basket. Add the remaining florets to the food processor and repeat, adding this batch now to the steamer. Add in 3/4 cup water to the pot and steam for 8 minutes.
- After steaming, the cauliflower will be HOT, so I like to spread it out on a plate to cool.
- Preheat the oven to 375 degrees
- After it has cooled, I use my nut milk bag to squeeze out ALL the water from the cauliflower. THIS STEP WILL MAKE OR BREAK THE TORTILLAS! You must squeeze all the water out as much as you can. I've found the less moisture, the better results.
- Add the cauliflower to a bowl. To the bowl also add in the eggs and spices. Mix well. It will look like a batter. Somewhat thick.
- Fit some parchment paper on top of two baking pans.
- Spoon the batter onto the parchment paper. I get about 6 out of this recipe, so three on each pan.

- The trick is to evenly spread the batter in a circle. Keep the batter compact. There should be no parchment showing through any area of the tortilla.
- Bake for 17 minutes. After they bake, I flip mine over and give them another 2 minutes.
- Remove from parchment and transfer to a cooling rack.

Notes:
*I prefer to make these earlier in the day. I store them in the fridge and simply heat on a pan before I serve.
*I cannot offer any subs for the eggs, as I've only made these with eggs.
*The cauliflower is not overwhelming and they don't taste too "eggy."

Chard Stem Pickles

It occurred to me that pickling would be a great thing to do with wide chard stalks. They're crunchy and absorbent, and the texture stands up to weeks of pickling. Red chard or a mix of rainbow chard stalks is especially pretty if you serve within a few days of pickling; in time, the color will fade. Slice them very thin.

1 to 2 cups very thinly sliced chard stalks (slice less than 1/4 inch thick)
1/2 cup seasoned rice wine vinegar
1 Tbsp. sherry vinegar
1/4 cup sugar
1 cup water
2 1/4 tsp. Himalayan salt

- Place the chard stalks in a jar or bowl.
- In a large bowl, combine the rice wine vinegar, sherry vinegar and sugar. Bring the water to a boil, remove from the heat and add to the vinegar and sugar mixture. Stir until the sugar is dissolved. Add the salt and stir well.
- Pour over the chard stalks, cover and refrigerate for at least 2 days before eating and for up to 2 weeks.

Shake the jar from time to time or, if you use a bowl, place a saucer on top of the chard stems to keep them submerged.

- Remove from the brine with a slotted spoon to serve.

Variation: Add to the chard stalks 4 small spring onions, bulbs only, cut in half lengthwise. This imparts a mild onion flavor to the brine and to the pickled chard stalks.

Advance preparation: These will stay crunchy and delicious for at least 10 days.

Pasta

There's increasing awareness of Celiac Disease, a serious allergy to wheat gluten that causes depression, early osteoarthritis, Irritable Bowel Syndrome, growth failure, autoimmune disease, abnormal liver function, poochy-belly, and a slew of avoidable health maladies. May I urge you to explore the new world of today's gluten-free pasta offerings. There are pastas made from quinoa, bean flour, brown rice, spelt, buckwheat, potato and rice flours, and on and on. Got wheat belly? Everyone should seriously consider cutting back on their consumption of wheat and wheat gluten. Today!

Fowler's House Pasta
Serves 4

1 pound of gluten-free pasta
½ cup EVOO
3 Tbsp. minced fresh garlic
2 cups chopped fresh tomatoes with skin
¼ cup capers with juice
1 bunch green onions, washed and chopped
2 oz. fresh basil leaves, washed and chopped
Himalayan salt and black pepper to taste
1 tsp. cayenne powder
¼ cup rice vinegar
½ cup nutritional yeast flakes or non-parmesan

- Cook and drain pasta according to package directions and keep warm.

- In a large sauté pan, heat the oil over medium heat and sauté garlic. Pull off the heat and add the tomatoes, capers, scallions, basil, salt and pepper, cayenne, and vinegar.
- In a large bowl, combine the cooked pasta and remaining garlic. Pour warm tomato mixture over the pasta and toss gently.
- Top with parmesan or nutritional yeast flakes and serve.

Sicilian Pasta

1 pound of pasta your choice (Quinoa, brown rice, rice, or bean flours)
4 Tbsp. EVOO
4 Tbsp. garlic, minced
½ tsp. black pepper
½ tsp. crushed red pepper
4 Tbsp. chopped cilantro
1 small can tomato concentrate
Salt to taste
Nutritional yeast flakes
Parmesan or appropriate substitute

- Cook pasta according to package instructions, Drain and keep warm.
- In a large sauté pan, warm the oil over medium-high heat. Add 2 Tbsp. of garlic, the black pepper, crushed red pepper, and tomato concentrate.
- Simmer 1 minute, stirring frequently with a wooden spoon.
- Twice, fill the empty tomato can with water, remove the resistant goodies remaining in the can, and then add it to the sauce. Blend.
- Reduce heat to low and simmer for 1 minute.

- Add the pasta, basil, and green onions to the sauce along with the remaining raw garlic. Mix gently and serve.
- Top with cheesy nutritional yeast flakes and chopped cilantro

Blissful Summer Soba Pho

This is a stress-free, fibrous, air-temp Asian noodle dish. Wasabi is made from a Japanese radish, with a bite similar to a very strong horseradish or Chinese mustard. Mix a small amount with water to make a thick green paste. Let it mature for five minutes to develop its full flavor. The burn is ephemeral, so don't worry about lingering heat. Actually, you'll probably want to blow your schnozzola after this dish, so it's a good expectorant that'll clear your sinus out in a jiffy.

Put your Pho ingredients into small bowls. Then create your soup by adding wasabi paste, ginger, bok choy and scallions to suit your taste. Each person puts their favorite additions in their empty bowl and then adds hot veggie stock to the tasty dish.

2 Tbsp. Wasabi powder (or commercially prepared paste)
1 Tbsp. salt-reduced, wheat-free soy sauce
1 Tbsp. Mirin
¼ cup fermented black bean paste
1 Tbsp. grated fresh ginger
4 slivered basil and mint leaves
1/4 cup scallions/green onions, finely cut
Thinly sliced bok choy
8 to 12 ounces buckwheat soba noodles
Assorted fresh chopped vegetables, thinly sliced
8 cups veggie stock
4 large soup bowls for serving

- Cook noodles according to package directions. Remove from heat and let sit for five minutes. Rinse and chill.

- In a small bowl, blend the wasabi power with 1 1/2 tsp. water and set aside for 5 minutes.
- To make the broth, in a large bowl mix the wasabi slurry into the wheat-free soy sauce, mirin, and fermented black bean paste. Add the 8 cups vegetable stock.
- Blend, then get the stock rip-roaring hot.
- To serve, place a portion of noodles, some chopped basil and mint, green onions, bok choy, and chopped vegetables equally into each large soup bowl.
- Moments before serving to your guests, carefully pour the boiling hot stock onto the patiently waiting ingredients. That's the only cooking it needs.
- Get your slurp on,

Vegan Pad Thai

An authentic Pad Thai recipe usually has tamarind juice or pulp to give it a distinct orange hue and sweet flavor. Tamarind can be hard to find depending on where you live. Try this easy vegetarian and vegan version instead.

1 pound Asian-style rice noodles
1/4 cup soy sauce
1/2 cup lime juice
2 Tbsp. peanut butter
2 Tbsp. hot sauce
1 Tbsp. Stevia powder
1 block tempeh, diced
1 onion, diced
4 cloves garlic, minced
2 Tbsp. Sesame oil
1/2 cup bean sprouts
1/4 cup chopped or crushed peanuts
4 green onions, sliced

- Cook noodles according to package instructions.
- Whisk together the soy sauce, peanut butter, lime juice,

hot sauce and stevia powder.

- In a large wok or skillet, sauté the tempeh, onion and garlic in sesame oil for a minute or two, stirring frequently. Allow to cook for another minute or two.
- To the cooked noodles add the peanut butter and soy sauce mixture. Stir well, and allow sauce to thicken as it cooks for about 3 minutes.
- Top with peanuts, bean sprouts and green onions and serve hot.

Summer Vegetables with Pasta
Serves 4

Mouthfuls of explosive flavor wait in the highly nutritious pasta dish that brims with protein and colorful fresh vegetable carbs: A veggie-licious entree that will increase your desire to consume more health-restoring, sun-blessed vegetables. You're doing great!

12 oz. Barilla plus spaghetti (or however much you think you need!)
1/2 green/red peppers, diced carrots, sliced red onions
3 garlic cloves minced
Basil, mint, and cilantro leaves, roughly torn
2Tbsp. ground flax or Chia seed (For fiber)
1 tsp. Himalayan salt
½ tsp. pepper flakes
2 Tbsp. chopped pecans or walnuts
Grated Parmesan

- Set a large pot of water on to boil. Add salt followed by the spaghetti. Cook al dente according to package instructions.
- Slice all the vegetables and mince the garlic. (Note: you can really put in any veg you like. It all works!)
- Heat the olive oil in a medium pan to medium heat. Add garlic and sauté for 1 minute. Add vegetables, then salt and hot pepper flakes. Stir constantly and watch the heat, cautious not to overcook.

- Drain the pasta, and add it to the warm vegetables. Combine all the ingredients.
- Plate the dish and sprinkle with the chopped nuts and grated parmesan.

Pasta with Spring Vegetables and a Tropical Twist

Celebrate the season of re-birth with a lean, clean waistline-friendly, spring vegetable and whole grain pasta dish.

8 ounce your favorite penne pasta
1 fake "chicken breast' cut into bite size slivers (Not made from wheat gluten)
2 Tbsp. unrefined raw virgin coconut oil
1 medium head garlic, minced
1 cup stewed tomatoes
1 large onion, chopped
2 Tbsp. ground flax seed
1/2 pound fresh asparagus
8 oz. sugar snap peas
1/2 cup beer
Himalayan salt and black pepper to taste
Chopped chives for garnish

- In a large pot cook with boiling salted water cook pasta until al dente. Drain.
- In a large skillet pan-fry the meat substitute in the coconut and half of the head of minced garlic until browned.
- Add the stewed tomatoes, the other half of the garlic, snow peas, asparagus and beer to a light boil.
- Shut off heat immediately and remove from burner. Don't over-cook the veggies.
- Toss in the cooked "meat" and ground flax seed.
- Toss pasta in with the garlic "meat" sauce.
- Garnish with chopped fresh chives.
- Serve warm.

Anti-inflammatory Tabbouleh with Quinoa
"Reconstructed"

½ cup washed quinoa seed
4 Tbsp. EVOO
3 cups vegetable stock
2 Tbsp. ground flax or chia seed
3 green onions, washed and chopped
3 garlic cloves, minced (Dry won't cut it)
3 cups washed, stemmed and finely chopped Kale
¾ cup mint, stemmed and chopped coarsely
4 tomatoes, diced
1 cucumber, skin on, diced
¼ cups lemon juice (Not from a bottle)
Himalayan salt and black pepper to taste

- Boil quinoa in water and olive oil for 10 minutes, pull off the fire, reserve and let reach room temperature. Do not overcook.
- Toss and fluff quinoa with all the remaining ingredients with a fork. Do not over mix and turn it into mush.
- Enjoy!!

Marinara Puttanesca in the Raw

2 fresh summer tomatoes, washed. Leave skin on-Vitamin C
1 cup sun-dried tomatoes, soaked in water for 10 minutes
2 cloves raw, peeled garlic
1 red bell pepper
1 Tbsp. fresh basil
2 tsp. fresh oregano
Kalamata olives, pitted and sliced
2 Tbsp. EVOO
¾ tsp. Sea salt
½ tsp. black pepper
1 dash cayenne
Gluten-free organic pasta
Non-parmesan cheese or nutritional yeast flakes

- Boil pasta based upon package instructions and reserve.

- Place all ingredients in food processor fitted with the S Blade.
- Let her rip!
- Top warm pasta with raw tomato sauce and crown with parmesan cheese.
- Serve over grilled fish and free-range chicken, too.

Pasta with Greens

1 bunch cooking greens (chard, collard greens, turnip greens, spinach)
1 Tbsp. Himalayan salt to taste
1 lb. your favorite non-wheat pasta
1 Tbsp. Nutritional yeast flakes
4 cloves garlic
2 Tbsp. EVOO
1/2 tsp. red pepper flakes
1 Tbsp. ground flax seeds
3/4 cups parmesan or nutritional yeast flakes

- Bring a large pot of water to a boil. Meanwhile, trim and wash the greens, leaving the leaves whole. Add 1 Tbsp. sea salt to the boiling water. Add greens and blanch for 30 seconds or until wilted.
- Use tongs or a slotted spoon to remove the leaves to a colander. In the same water, boil pasta until tender to the bite.
- Drain, reserved 1/2 cup of the cooking liquid, and set aside.
- Meanwhile, chop garlic and cooked greens.
- Once pasta is drained, return pot to medium-high heat. Add oil, garlic, pepper flakes. Cook stirring, until garlic turns just the tiniest bit golden
- Add chopped greens, yeast and flax. Stir to combine. Add reserved liquid and bring to a boil. Add pasta, stir to combine, and bring to a boil. Take off heat. Stir in half of the 'cheese'. Taste and add salt to taste.
- Divide between plates or pasta bowls, garnish with remaining "cheese," and serve.

Creamy Pacific Garden Pasta Salad

10 Side Dish Servings
Get ready for a screaming food-gasm!!!

1# box your favorite pasta
1/3 cup Veganese mayo
1/3 cup coconut milk, the heavy cream of South East Asia
2 Tbsp. coconut oil
1 Tbsp. fresh lime juice
1 Tbsp. raw local honey
1 clove garlic, minced
1/8 tsp. Himalayan salt
Black pepper to taste
1 cup halved cherry or grape tomatoes
1 cup diced green pepper
1 cup grated carrots (2 carrots)
½ cup chopped macadamia nuts
½ cup shredded coconut flakes, unsweetened

Garnish:
1 Tbsp. fresh basil
1 Tbsp. cup chopped green onions
1 tsp. macadamia nuts, chopped

- Cook pasta "al dente" in pot of boiling salted water, around 10 minutes or follow package instructions. Drain and refresh under cold running water.
- Whisk mayonnaise, coconut milk and oil, vinegar, lime juice, honey, garlic, salt and pepper in a large bowl until smooth.
- Add the cooked pasta and gently stir to coat, not too aggressively or it will break up the pasta.
- Add vegetables, nuts, coconut flakes and gently stir.
- Serve and garnish individual portions with basil, nuts and green onions.

Cinnamon-Lime Dressing

¼ Cup EVOO
1 lime, juiced
1 Tbsp. Bragg's apple cider vinegar
¼ tsp. Himalayan salt
1/8 tsp. cinnamon
1/8 tsp. grated, fresh ginger

- Place all of the ingredients in a small bowl and whisk to combine.
- Add to your salad and toss to combine

Entrees

Vegan Sweet Potato Hash

Always scrub your spud and produce to remove field residue and any, ahem, poo, left by a passing critter. In this recipe we bake the root tuber first. Sweet potatoes are loaded with vitamins C, A, and colon cleansing fiber.

2 medium, pre-baked sweet potatoes cubed. (Skins on)
1 green pepper, coarsely chopped
½ onion, coarsely chopped
¼ fresh jalapeno pepper, finely chopped
2 garlic cloves, finely chopped
1 Tbsp. potato starch
¼ tsp. red pepper or chipotle flakes

- Lightly oil a large sauté pan over medium heat.
- In a mixing bowl, toss in the cooked, cooled potatoes, jalapeno, green pepper, garlic and chipotle and mix gently. We don't want mashed potatoes.
- Wet your hands and form uniform patties in your palm.
- Place them in the awaiting sauté pan. Be patient and only turn them once or they'll break up.

- Wait until one side is browned and crispy before flipping. Too much handling is not cool.

Israeli Falafel
Serves 4

1-15 ounce can of garbanzo beans, drained or 1 pound cooked from dry
½ cup of chopped onion
¼ cup bread crumbs
1 Tbsp. chopped parsley
1 tsp. cumin powder
½ tsp. coriander
¼ tsp. Himalayan salt
1/8 tsp. each, black and cayenne pepper
2 Cloves of chopped, fresh, garlic
2 tsp. EVOO, divided

Tahini Sauce:
1 jar of Tahini sauce (made from sesame seeds)
Water or vegetable stock to thin
2 Tbsp. lemon juice

- Place 6 Tbsp. of Tahini in a small mixing bowl. A little at a time, whisk lemon juice and water until the sauce has thinned out, a bit like syrup.

Patties:
- Add the first 20 ingredients to a food processor and process until smooth.
- Divide the mixture into 8 patties, or 16 smaller appetizer size for a lovely cocktail party hors d'oeuvres.
- Coat a large non-stick skillet with Pam spray, and add one teaspoon of olive oil and place the pan over medium heat. Cook approximately 4 minutes on each side until golden brown.

- Repeat the procedure with the remaining oil and patties.
- Eat the crispy critters immediately and then pour on the Tahini sauce for a truly classical Israeli food.
- Cilantro pesto also adds to the nutrient value of this classic dish.

Cilantro Pesto

1 clove of garlic
1/2 cup of almonds, cashews, or other nuts
1 cup packed fresh cilantro leaves, washed to remove field residue
2 Tbsp. Lemon juice
6 Tbsp. EVOO

- Place everything into a food processer and let 'er rip.

Ayurveda Kitchari

Kitchari is an easy-to-digest, traditional healing rice and bean dish; the comfort food of India. In this recipe we use the heavy cream of the Orient, delicious, creamy coconut milk and healing coconut oil.

1 cup split yellow mung dal / moong dahl, or red lentils
2 cups cooked Indian or California long grain basmati rice (Quinoa would work fine too.)
1 cup chopped almonds
3 Tbsp. organic, ghee or unrefined virgin coconut oil
2 Tbsp. coconut milk
1 inch piece of fresh ginger root, peeled, chopped well
1 tsp. caraway seed
1 tsp. fennel seed
1 tsp. cumin seed
1 tsp. cinnamon
Pinch of cayenne
½ tsp. turmeric
1 cup assorted, washed veggies: peas, carrots, cauliflower, red peppers, zucchini.

(Keep shape uniform so things will cook evenly)
Cilantro leaves for garnish
2 bunches chopped green onions for garnish

- First, wash and rinse the mung dal and rice. In a sauce pan, heat 9 cups of water until it boils; add the mung dahl and rice. Stir and cover and cook for 25 minutes.
- Crush the fennel, caraway, and cumin. In another pan, heat the ghee or coconut oil on medium and add the ginger, seeds, turmeric, cayenne, turmeric, cinnamon sticks. It should smell heavenly by now! If you are adding veggies, add them to the spices once the spices are roasted.
- Over medium-low heat, briefly sauté the vegetables being sure not to overcook. You'll destroy the vitamins and digestive enzymes if you do.
- Add the rice, dal and coconut milk, and then gently mix. Do not over mix and turn this into mush.
- Garnish with chopped almonds, green onion, and cilantro.

Sweet and Savory Fruited Barley Pilaf
8 servings

3/4 cup pearl barley
2-1/4 cups water
1 cup chopped onion
2 to 3 cloves garlic, finely chopped
1 cup chopped Granny Smith apple
1 cup (6 ounces) dried apricots, snipped into 1/2-inch pieces
1/3 cup organic, no-sugar-added, orange marmalade
2 tsp. grated fresh lemon peel
2 Tbsp. fresh lemon juice
2 Tbsp. orange juice
1 tsp. Himalayan salt
1/2 tsp. dried or fresh leaf oregano
1/2 tsp. dried or fresh thyme
1/4 tsp. ground white pepper

- In medium saucepan with lid, bring water to a boil. Add barley and return to boil. Reduce heat to low, cover and cook 45 minutes or until Barley is tender and liquid is absorbed.
- Set aside. Spray large skillet with non-stick cooking spray. Sauté onion and garlic for 5 minutes, stirring occasionally.
- Mix in apple and apricots. Sauté 3 more minutes.
- Blend in marmalade, lemon peel, lemon juice, orange juice, salt, oregano, thyme and white pepper. Simmer for 5 minutes, stirring occasionally.
- Add barley, cook 5 minutes longer.
- Enjoy.

Summer Vegetable Paella
Serves 6 to 8

Chef Wendell continues his quest to encourage vegaphobic Earthlings to eat more nutritious, fibrous vegetables. You don't have to make this vegetable-rich dish in a paella pan. Serve as a main or side dish.

1 quart vegetable stock
Generous pinch (about 1/2 teaspoon) saffron threads or 1 tsp. turmeric
2 cups long grain basmati white rice
2 Tbsp. EVOO
1 medium onion, finely chopped
4 large garlic cloves, minced
1 red pepper, cut into strips
1 green pepper, cut into strips
1 Tbsp. tomato paste
1 tsp. sweet paprika
1 pound ripe tomatoes, or 1- 14-ounce can chopped tomatoes with juice
1/4 pound green beans, trimmed and cut in 1-inch lengths

1 can chickpeas, drained and rinsed, or 1 1/2 cups fresh or frozen Lima beans
1 cup frozen peas
Himalayan salt and freshly ground pepper

- Bring the stock to a simmer in a medium saucepan. Crush the saffron threads between your fingertips, and place in a small bowl. Add 1 tablespoon warm water, and set aside.
- Heat the oil over medium heat in a large, heavy frying pan or a paella pan. Add the onion. Cook, stirring, until the onion is tender, about three minutes. Add the garlic, peppers and a generous pinch of salt.
- Cook, stirring, until the peppers begin to soften, about one minute. Add the tomato paste, paprika and rice. Cook, stirring, for 1 minute until the grains begin to crackle. Add the tomatoes and cook, stirring, until they cook down slightly and smell fragrant, about 5 minutes.
- Stir in the saffron or turmeric with its soaking water, scraping in every last bit with a rubber spatula. Season generously with salt and pepper.
- Add stock, green beans and chickpeas or lima beans. Bring to a boil. Stir once, reduce the heat to medium-low, and simmer without stirring until the liquid has just about evaporated, about 10 to 15 minutes. Add the peas. Continue to simmer until the rice is dry, another 5 to 10 minutes.
- Remove from the heat and serve.

Chickpea Cutlets

2 cups cooked (or canned) beans, mashed
2 Tbsp. EVOO
Up to 1 cup of gluten-free breadcrumbs

4 Tbsp. ground flax
3 Tbsp. wheat-free tamari
2 cloves garlic, crushed
1 tsp. paprika
1 tsp. onion powder
½ tsp. lemon zest
½ tsp. Himalayan salt (optional)
1 cup of coarse flour (chickpea, rice, or gluten-free flour to coat)
Expeller-pressed cooking oil for gentle frying and browning

Optional: add more chickpea flour if mix is too wet.

- Mix everything together (except the coarse gluten-free flour, chickpea flour, and cooking oil) in a big, round-sided mixing bowl.
- The mix should stick together well, but not be too wet. Needs to be borderline wet-sticky, so they won't fall apart when cooking. If the mix is too wet, add chickpea flour until you're satisfied.
- Form into patties or cutlet shapes – whatever floats your boat.
- Coat each patty with a layer of coarse gluten-free flour.
- Pan-fry in cooking oil on med-high heat until toasty on the outside, then drain on paper towels, or brush patties with oil and bake on an oiled/lined tray at 350°F until the outside is nicely browned. (If you're worried about cutlets falling apart, the oven bake is your best bet!)

"Raw" Mushroom Pizza

1 large Portobello mushroom, washed and dried with flutes removed with teaspoon
Juice of one lemon
¼ cup raw tahini or almond paste
¼ avocados, peeled, pitted, and thinly sliced
½ ripe tomato, sliced thin
1 Tbsp. EVOO

4 tsp. ground flax seed
Himalayan salt and black pepper to taste

- Remove and discard the stem of the shroom and remove the mushroom cap "gills" with a tablespoon.
- Turn cap upside down and place on a serving plate. Sprinkle 1 tsp. of flax seed per pizza.
- Squeeze fresh lemon juice over it and then spoon in the tahini.
- Top with sliced tomatoes and avocado.
- Season with sea salt and pepper. Drizzle with extra virgin olive oil
- Cut into quarters and serve.

Warm Quinoa Pilaf with fresh Cranberry and Almonds
Serves 6

When the joyous holidays hit, we naturally lose our human resolve and overeat. By including more fiber in the festive foods, you can reduce the damage. As always, I suggest ground flax seed with Omega-3 EFA's seeds sprinkled on each dish to lessen the arterial carnage. I promise it disappears; no one will see it. But the ground seed creates a slurry, and acts like Roto-Rooter, reducing the time the dead animal gravy rots in your digestive track where it's uploaded into your arteries.

Plus, if you have a vegetarian or Celiac coming for Thanksgiving, they will give thanks for this tasty, gluten and wheat-free side dish. Fibrous Quinoa is naturally wheat and gluten-free and is a complete protein for vegans and vegetarians. Try this quick, flavorful pilaf.

1 Tbsp. extra-virgin olive oil
1 Small red onion, chopped
1 Tbsp. orange zest
1 Tbsp. real maple syrup, honey, or stevia powder
1 cup fresh, washed cranberries
1 stick diced celery
1 carrot, diced
1 cup uncooked quinoa, rinsed and drained

2 cups vegetable broth
1/2 tsp. Himalayan salt
2/3 cup sliced almonds, toasted

- Cook quinoa per instructions, but in veggie stock, not plain water. Drain.
- Heat oil in a medium pot over medium-high heat. Add onions, carrots, cranberry, and celery and cook, stirring often, until just softened. (2 minutes).
- Add cooked quinoa and sweetener of choice; toss and mix for 1 minute.
- Garnish with chopped almonds and orange zest then serve.

Quinoa Pilaf with Chai Cherries and Walnuts

¾ cup quinoa, rinsed well
2 Tbsp. EVOO
2 stalks chopped celery
3 green onions, thinly sliced
2 ½ cups veggie stock
¾ tsp. Himalayan salt
¼ tsp. black pepper
1/3 cup dried cherries or cranberries
1 cup stout, brewed chai tea
¼ cup chopped raw walnuts or almonds

- Place quinoa seed in a colander and rinse under cold running water. Drain well.
- Rehydrate the cherries in warm chai tea. Reserve juice.
- In a large skillet, heat oil over medium.
- Add scallions and garlic and cook, stirring often for 2 minutes or until scallions are barely tender.
- Stir in the quinoa and cook 2-3 minutes or until lightly toasted.
- Add boiling vegetable stock, salt and pepper.

- Reduce to a simmer, cover and cook 10 to 15 minutes or until quinoa's little tail pops out.
- Stir in the nuts, drained cherries and just a bit of the reserved juice.
- Don't add to much chai juice or the dish with become soupy.

Sweet Potato and Spinach Hash

You should eat sweet potatoes, a super food more often than just at Thanksgiving. They're packed with beta-carotene, an antioxidant that fights aging. You eat to gain energy, lower your cholesterol level, maintain digestive health and, of course, to help create gorgeous skin. Pack all four of these benefits into one awesome dish. Plus, it only takes minutes to make.

1/2 cup onion, finely chopped
1 clove garlic, minced
2 tbsp. EVOO
1 sweet potato, small dice (about 2 cups)
2 large local eggs, mixed with fork
Several drops liquid smoke
1 tsp. dried thyme
Himalayan salt and pepper to taste
1 tsp. cumin
1/2 tsp. chili powder
1/2 tsp. ground coriander
5 oz. chopped fresh spinach (about 2 cups packed)
¼ cups walnut pieces
1/4 cup water
Chopped fresh parsley for garnish

- Heat oil in skillet over medium heat. Add onions and garlic and sauté 1 minute. Add sweet potatoes, eggs and seasonings. Cook, stirring occasionally, until potatoes are just tender but still firm in the middle.
- Stir in liquid smoke and cook about a minute, then add spinach and cook until it just starts to wilt. (About 2 minutes).

- Using large spatula, transfer pile of hash to each serving plates. Garnish with parsley and serve.

Spinach

This leafy green vegetable is rich in nutrients and antioxidants. Spinach is loaded with lutein, which keeps your eyes healthy and sparkling. Spinach is also a good source of vitamins B, C, and E, potassium, calcium, iron, magnesium, and Omega-3 fatty acids. Trade your lettuce for spinach, or sauté spinach for a quick, healthy side.

Walnuts

You don't need to eat cupfuls of walnuts to enjoy their many benefits: smoother skin, healthy hair, brighter eyes, and strong bones. Get your daily dose of nutrients like Omega-3 fatty acids and vitamin E by eating a handful by themselves or throwing some in your salad, pasta, or dessert.

Roasted Sweet Potato Taco with Black Beans

4 medium sweet potatoes scrubbed, washed, and cut into ½ inch cubes
1 large onion
½ cup extra virgin olive oil
Himalayan salt and cracked black keeper to taste
1 tsp. minced fresh hot chili pepper
1 garlic clove, minced
Juice of 2 limes
2 cups cooked and rinsed black beans
1 red and 1 yellow pepper seeded and cut into ¼ inch dice pieces
1 cup fresh chopped cilantro
1 head romaine or bib lettuce washed and pat dry (select broad leaves)

- Pre-heat oven to 400˚.

- Cut the potatoes into cubes; do not remove skin.
- Put potato and onion in a mixing bowl and drizzle with 2 Tbsp. extra virgin oil. Toss and spread in single layer onto a sheet pan. Sprinkle with salt and pepper.
- Roast for 20 minutes turning with a spatula often.
- Place potatoes in mixing bowl and add the drained black beans and gently mix
- In a blender or food processer, blend the chili, garlic, and lime, salt and pepper. While potatoes are still warm, toss everything together gently.
- Place a tablespoon or more of the sweet potato mix at the bottom of the lettuce rib. Roll up from the bottom like you would a burrito or egg roll. (The envelope fold).
- Place on serving platter seam side down, drizzle with more lime juice. Serve at room temperature.

Ghoulish Goulash

Parents, there are ghoulish dangers awaiting your children on Halloween – scary dangers like high-fructose corn syrup, sugar, refined carbohydrates, food coloring, artificial flavorings, trans fats, and triglycerides, just to name a spooky few. All of these kick the "BOO" out of your immune system leaving the door ajar for flu.

All of these common ingredients in Halloween candy are linked to such conditions as childhood obesity, coronary artery disease, diabetes, yeast overgrowth syndrome and multiple-chemical sensitivity. *Very frightening!!* If you find this hauntingly objectionable, serve this vegetable rich goulash to neutralize the damage. "Over-dosing on sugar, is very hard on your pancreas". Sugar is a proven, toxic drug, friends. Too much of anything is not good. The vegetables and fiber in this dish will help neutralize the damage from the annual Halloween sugar bloodbath of sugary gore. This year I'm handing out insulin.

1 tsp. EVOO
½ medium onion, sliced thin
1 carrot, chopped
¼ cup celery
2 cloves of chopped garlic
1 cup shiitake mushrooms, sliced thin stems discarded
1 green pepper, sliced thin
1 Tbsp. ground flax seeds
½ cup 'meat' crumbles
1 tsp. paprika
1-14 ½ oz. can whole canned tomatoes, chopped, reserve juice
1 cup of cooked beans, drained
½ cup red wine vinegar
1 tsp. oregano

- Heat the olive oil over medium heat.
- Sautee the onion, celery, peppers, carrot, garlic, paprika, meat crumbles and mushrooms until just tender.
- Stir in the tomatoes with juice. Add beans, wine, oregano and reserved tomato juice.
- Bring to a boil, but do not cook more than 3 minutes. Add flax and stir.
- Serve over a bed of brown rice, whole wheat pasta or quinoa and a dark leafy green salad.

Braised Moroccan Eggplant with Garbanzo Beans

1 onion, sliced thin
5 cloves of chopped, fresh garlic
1 red bell pepper, cut into 1" cubes
1 medium eggplant, cut into 1 inch cubes
Pinch of red pepper flakes
½ tsp. Garam masala or curry powder
1-15 oz. can garbanzo beans, drained
2 cups cooked lentils, drained
½ cup tomato sauce
1/2 cups vegetable broth / stock
½ cup raisins
1 Tbsp. chopped fresh cilantro
Himalayan salt and cracked black pepper to taste

- Chop garlic and onion and let sit for 5 minutes to bring out their health promoting properties.
- Into a skillet, add 1 Tbsp. of the vegetable stock.
- Heat to medium; add the onions and garlic, red pepper, chili flakes, raisins, eggplant, masala, and turmeric.
- Sauté 3 minutes.
- Add broth and tomato sauce.
- Stir occasionally until the eggplant and peppers are just tender. Don't overcook, please.
- Add the garbanzos and lentils. Bring to a simmer and shut off the heat.
- Serve and top with chopped cilantro.
- Serve with quinoa, brown rice, barley and a dark-green leafy vegetable salad.

Asian Pumpkin Stir-Fry

There are many reasons pumpkin should be eaten, just like squash, year around, or at least in season. Pumpkin flesh is exceptionally high in carotenoids that give pumpkins their orange colors. Carotenoids are really good at neutralizing naughty free radicals, malicious molecules that can attack cell membranes and leave the cells susceptible to damage. One pound of 'fresh' pumpkin, diced (a small pie pumpkin or Jack-o-lantern entrails).

2 organic local eggs
2 stalks of celery, chopped
4 stalks of green onions, chopped
1 red pepper, chopped coarse
1 Tbsp. chopped cilantro
½ onion, sliced
1 pkg. Stevia
Water
3 garlic cloves, chopped
2 Tbsp. wheat-free soy sauce
2 Tbsp. oyster sauce (Optional)
1 Tbsp. fish sauce (Optional)
¼ tsp. black pepper
3 Tbsp. expeller-pressed peanut or safflower oil

- Peel and cut the pumpkin (canned pumpkin will turn to mush)
- Over medium-high heat, add the garlic and oil to a non-corrosive sauté pan to release the flavors.
- Add the egg and stir-fry until half cooked.
- Add the pumpkin, spring onion, pepper, celery, onions, water, fish sauce, oyster sauce, Stevia, soy sauce and pepper. Everything but the cilantro.
- Stir fry for 1 minute.
- Plate and garnish with cilantro leaves.

Jamaican Coconut Rice and Beans
Serves: 4-5

1 medium sized can organic red kidney beans
1 can unsweetened coconut milk (shake well)
2 cups of long-grain brown rice
2 green onions, chopped
1 Tbsp. ground flax seeds
1 clove garlic, chopped
1 Tbsp. fresh thyme
2 Tbsp. organic, unrefined coconut oil
1 Scotch bonnet pepper (whole, do not chop up) or jalapeno, Serrano or your favorite pepper

- Drain the liquid from the can of beans.
- Over medium heat, cook 2 cups of the brown rice in 5 cups of water and 1 cup of coconut milk.
- Place the whole scotch bonnet pepper on top of the rice and boil for 20 minutes. Turn off the heat, and place a lid on the pot.
- Meanwhile, place the beans, onions, garlic, thyme and coconut oil in a sauté pan over med-low heat, stirring.
- Remove scotch bonnet or other pepper used from pot and add to bean mixture, mixing thoroughly.
- Serve warm.

Cajun Beans and Rice

1 Tbsp. expeller pressed vegetable oil
1/2 pound "FAKE" meat sausage, sliced into 1/2 inch thick
slices
1 medium onion, chopped
1 medium green bell pepper, chopped
2 cloves garlic, minced
6 cups cooked brown rice
1 can kidney beans, drained and rinsed
1 can navy beans, drained and rinsed
3-1/2 cups canned stewed tomatoes, Cajun-style
Fresh chopped oregano leaves
1 tsp. dijon
1/2 tsp. tabasco
1 cup green onions, thinly sliced

- Heat oil in large skillet over medium-high heat until hot. Add "sausage," onion, green pepper and garlic.
- Cook, stirring 7-10 minutes, or until meat is browned and onion is tender.
- Add rice, kidney beans, navy beans, stewed tomatoes, oregano, dijon and hot sauce.
- Cook and stir 2-3 minutes more until well-blended and thoroughly heated. Sprinkle with green onions and oregano and then serve immediately.

Gorp
4 Servings

This is a remarkably satisfying and filling vegetarian dish the whole family will love. Smaller red bliss potatoes have a lower glycemic load.

1 pound organic baby red or Yukon gold potatoes, boiled with skin on
2 cups cooked brown rice or quinoa
1/2 Pound chopped, cooked spinach, chard, or dark leafy greens drained
1 chopped onion
1 grated carrot
2 Tbsp. ground flax seeds

6 oz. organic silken tofu
Himalayan salt and black pepper to taste
Warm organic vegetable stock

- Wash your spuds then boil them until just done. Use a fork to test doneness.
- While still warm, mash the potatoes with the rice and the remaining ingredients until the desired consistency is achieved. Leave them a little chunky and try your best not to over whip.

Mediterranean Bean Salad

Economical beans, the poor man's meat, were one of the first cultivated crops and are intricately woven into the tapestry of human history. Early evidence of bean consumption dates back to 9750 BC.
Legumes are an essential part of a balanced vegan diet. Beans, grains, nuts, and seeds have a symbiotic relationship in which the combined amino acids of each form complete plant proteins, the foundation for growth and development of life. Vitamins B1 and B2 can be found kidney beans.
If the after-effects of eating beans are an issue, get over it! You should be more worried about the exhaust coming from your car, not your, ahem...well, I think you know where I'm going. Buy some Beano, and air-freshener for goodness sakes. Beans are one of the richest sources of fiber that prevents many diseases of the GI tract. Let's call fiber the "Colon-Pow!" of your GI tract. If you are burned out on fatty, highly-caloric, oily mayonnaise based bean salads, this salads delivers.

1/3 cup fresh lemon juice
2 Tbsp. EVOO
½ tsp. Himalayan salt
½ tsp. black pepper
½ tsp. paprika
¼ tsp. pepper flakes
½ cup chopped walnuts or almonds
1 can red kidney beans, drained and rinsed
1 can cannellini beans, drained and rinsed
¾ cup chopped red onion or scallion

12 oz. grape tomatoes cut in half
1/2 cup chopped fresh parsley or oregano

- Simply mix all ingredients together in a mixing bowl, refrigerate then serve.
- Serve with a salad of dark leafy greens, olive oil, garlic and mild vinegar.

Boraccho Beans
(Drunken Beans)

Archaeologists in Thailand found evidence of legume cultivation carbon dated to 9750 BC. The people of Mexico and Peru were cultivating bean crops as far back as 7000 BC. Regular consumption of fibrous foods is associated with a reduction in the risk of coronary heart disease. A high-fiber diet, particularly one high in water-soluble fiber (as in legumes), is associated with decreased risk of both fatal and nonfatal heart attacks, probably because fiber is known to lower cholesterol.

1 Tbsp. EVOO
½ onion, chopped
1 stalk celery, chopped
½ green bell pepper
1 carrot, diced
1 cup local corn
½ Jalapeno pepper, seeded and chopped
2 cloves of minced, fresh garlic
1 tsp. chili powder
1 tsp. cumin
1 tsp. cinnamon
1 tomato, chopped
1/8 Tbsp. Liquid smoke
2 Tbsp. crumbled tempeh drizzled with liquid smoke
2 pounds cooked pinto or black beans, drained
1 cup beer
Himalayan salt and pepper to taste
1 cup chopped fresh cilantro

- Heat olive oil in a sauté pan over medium heat. Add cumin and chili powder.

- Add the onion, corn, celery, jalapeno, green pepper, carrot, and crumbled "smoked" tempeh and garlic then sauté over medium-high for 1 minute.
- Add the drained beans and beer to the pan and simmer. Stir frequently with a wooden spoon.
- Eat!

Basic Vegetable Stir-Fry
With Tempeh and Almonds

The stir-fry process happens quickly, so be prepared. Have the slurry, vegetables, and tempeh ready to roll. I suggest using a wooden spoon.

¼ cup low-sodium, wheat-free soy sauce, plus 2 Tbsp. divided
2 tsp. raw honey
2 Tbsp. Mirin
1 block tempeh, cubed
1 tsp. chopped green onions
¼ tsp. fresh grated ginger
1 hot pepper, minced
1 cup small diced tempeh cubes-protein and fiber
1 tsp. potato flour instead of cornstarch
3 Tbsp. expeller pressed peanut oil
3 cups assorted vegetables: peppers, bok choy, broccoli, zucchini, carrot, snow or sugar snap peas
3 cups long-grain brown rice, Indian or California basmati, or quinoa
4 Tbsp. chopped almonds
4 tsp. ground flax or chia seed

- In a small bowl, mix the soy sauce, 1 tsp. honey, 1 Tbsp. Mirin, scallion and ginger.
- Add cubed tempeh and marinate for 15 minutes minimum.
- Remove the tempeh and reserve the liquid.
- Make slurry. Take remaining soy, 1 tsp. honey and mix in with the potato starch. Blend until all is dissolved.

- Heat pan very hot. Add 1 Tbsp. oil and quickly brown the tempeh and hot pepper. Remove and set aside.
- Using small amounts of oil, stir-fry the veggies – a few at a time please. If you overcrowd, you'll steam them! Cook in small batches if necessary starting with those that take the longest. Transfer cooked veggies to a covered dish.
- When all the veggies are tender yet al dente, add back to the pan along with tempeh.
- Stir in sauce / slurry and stir constantly until thickened. If too thick, thin with veggie stock or the reserved marinating sauce you made earlier.
- Garnish each serving with a tablespoon of almonds and ground flax seed, and serve promptly over rice, quinoa, alternative noodles.

Corn and Tomato Polenta with Oregano Pesto

1 qt. vegetable stock
1/4 tsp. Himalayan salt
1 cup yellow organic, non GMO - local cornmeal
1/2 cup Eden brand tomato sauce (No BPA in their cans)
1/2 cup whole-kernel organic corn, drained
Pepper to taste

Garnish:
1 bunch fresh oregano
¼ cup EVOO
Himalayan salt and pepper to taste

- In a heavy, 3-quart saucepan, bring stock and sea salt to a boil. Slowly pour cornmeal into a saucepan so the stock doesn't stop boiling, stirring to keep smooth and from scorching on the bottom.

- Reduce heat and simmer 20 minutes, stirring often until mixture is stiff.
- In between, grab your blender and toss in the oregano and olive oil. Puree.
- Meanwhile, in a small saucepan, heat tomato sauce, corn, cayenne, and pepper.
- When cornmeal is stiff, turn half into a serving dish and top with half the sauce.
- Layer remaining cornmeal and sauce and let rest 5 to 10 minutes.
- Cut in squares, top with 1 Tbsp. oregano pesto and serve proudly.

Colcannon
3 large or 4 medium servings

A traditional, old-world dish composed of creamed kale, leeks, and potatoes.

4 medium or 3 large potatoes
3½ cup chopped kale (one bunch)*
3 Leeks, washed
1 onion
1/3 cup almond or rice milk
¼ cup fresh parsley, chopped
Himalayan salt and freshly ground pepper to taste

- Cut up the potatoes and steam until soft. Meanwhile, chop the onion and sauté in a non-stick pan with a little water (no oil).
- Take a leek, *pause*, wash and trim, then cut into ½ inch pieces.
- Chop and wash the kale, and when the onion is soft, add the kale and leeks to the skillet; cover and let steam in the water that stays on the leaves after washing.
- When the potatoes are done, drain if necessary and mash with the skin. Mix in the almond or rice milk, parsley, and salt and pepper to taste: combine with the kale, leeks and serve.

*If kale is hard to find, most greens like mustard, turnip, collard, bok choy can be used. Green or red cabbage is also a traditional colcannon ingredient.

Twisted Sheppard's Pie

This is a satisfying rib-sticker bursting with wholesome nutrition. We've "greened-up" this timeless classic by removing the artery-detonating cholesterol so our heart patient friends can enjoy it, too. We left in the full-bodied flavor, however, leaving a tasty comfort food to warm yourself during these long winter days.

Mashed potato topping (Make this first):
2 Large potatoes, scrubbed and washed
1 Tbsp. EVOO
1/2 cup plain almond or coconut milk
3 large cloves garlic, minced
Himalayan salt and pepper to taste
1/2 cup minced fresh parsley

- Cut potatoes into chunks and boil until fork tender. Drain and keep warm.
- Add remaining ingredients and mash potatoes in traditional fashion.

Vegetable Hash:
1 Tbsp. EVOO
1 1/2 cups minced onions
4 Large cloves garlic, minced
1 tsp. Sea salt
2 Tbsp. ground flax or chia seeds
Fresh black pepper to taste
1 stalk celery, finely minced
1 lb. cremini or shiitake mushrooms, chopped
1 lb. zucchini, diced
1 medium bell pepper, minced
2 tsp. dried basil
1/2 tsp. dried thyme
1/2 tsp. dried oregano
1 cup peas (fresh or frozen)
3/4 cup grated non-dairy cheddar cheese

Cayenne to taste
Paprika
1 pound Yukon Gold potatoes
Almond milk

To make the vegetable hash and assembly:

- Preheat oven to 350°. Have a 2-quart casserole or a 9 x13 baking pan ready.
- Heat the oil in a large, deep skillet. Add the onion and sauté over medium heat for about 3 minutes, or until it begins to soften.
- Add garlic, salt, pepper, celery, mushrooms, zucchini and bell pepper. Stir until well combined, cover. Cook over medium heat for about 8 minutes, stirring frequently. Add the herbs, stir, and cover again. Cook for about 3 more minutes, or until the zucchini is al dente. Remove from heat.
- Stir in the peas and cheese. Add cayenne to taste. Transfer this mixture to the casserole or baking pan and spread it out.
- Spoon and/or spread the mashed potatoes over the vegetables. Dust generously with paprika.
- Bake uncovered for 10 minutes.
- Dig in.

Puerto Rican Peas and Rice
6 Main Dishes

Sandi and I reduced the waistline-expanding saturated fats in the traditional dish by omitting the lard and bacon. Flavor is not lost as we simply substitute the smoky flavor with liquid smoke. No one will know the difference unless you make an announcement. Let the families eat it, compliment it, and then you can let them know the secret: Got to be lovingly sneaky sometimes.

2 pounds fresh or frozen Peas
6 drops of liquid smoke to replace bacon

Eat Right Now

1 chopped onion
3 cloves of chopped garlic
1 chopped green pepper
8 oz. tomato sauce
1 Tbsp. turmeric
1 cup frozen peas
1 ½ tsp. Himalayan salt and pepper to taste
4 cups of HOT cooked, long grain Basmati rice
Fresh oregano leaves, chopped

- Over medium heat, sauté the onions, green pepper, turmeric, and garlic in olive or peanut oil. Stir occasionally.
- Drain the peas.
- Add salt and pepper to taste. Serve over rice and garnish with chopped oregano leaves.

Ratatouille
a spectacular, simple stew, soup or side dish

4 small zucchini
2 medium eggplants (do not peel)
4 ripe tomatoes, washed
1 green pepper
1 onion
2 cloves chopped garlic
1 bunch of parsley, chopped
EVOO
1 cup of pitted Greek or Nicoise' olives
Himalayan salt and pepper
1 tsp. dry thyme

- Cut all vegetables into 1 inch cubes. Keep vegetables separate. The order of cooking is important.
- Sauté the onion, garlic and peppers in olive oil over a brisk heat, Stirring frequently. Season with salt and pepper to taste.
- When the peppers are three-fourths cooked and still crunchy, pull them off the

fire and remove them from the pan.

- In the same fashion, sauté the eggplant until it is cooked through and golden. Set it aside with the peppers to keep each other company.
- Next sauté the thyme and zucchini until they are brown.
- Add the olives, tomatoes and parsley, and cook for an additional 2-3 minutes. Don't forget to stir!
- Return peppers and zucchini and mix the veggies thoroughly and serve.

Coconut Garbanzo Bean Curry

2 Tbsp. unrefined, virgin coconut oil
1 medium onion, diced
2 small-medium potatoes, diced
1 large or 2 small carrots, diced
1 can garbanzo beans, rinsed and drained well
1/2 cup water
2 tsp. green curry paste
1/4-1/2 cup coconut milk
1 tsp. garam masala
1-2 tsp. cumin
2 tsp. fresh ginger, peeled and minced
2-3 cloves garlic
Fresh black pepper and salt to taste
Fresh mint, about a handful, chopped

- Heat oil in large skillet and add the onion. Cook until translucent.
- Add garlic and ginger and cook for another minute or so.
- Add water, potatoes and carrots, and let simmer until veggies are tender and the water has boiled away.
- Add the garbanzo beans and the rest of the spices, including the curry paste. Add the coconut milk. It will seem runny at first, but let it simmer until it reaches desired consistency.

- Add the mint leaves at the end. Serve over a bed of brown rice, quinoa, or as a soup.

Wine Braised Lentils

3/4 cup green lentils
4 tsp. EVOO
1/3 cup each diced onions, carrot and celery
2 garlic cloves, 1 crushed, 1 halved
1 Tbsp. tomato paste
1 ½ cups dry red wine
1 tsp. Dijon
Himalayan salt and freshly ground pepper
12 pearl onions
1 big bunch of washed spinach or other greens such as stemmed kale leaves
1 tsp. expeller-pressed walnut or vegetable oil
4 slices Ezekiel, non-gluten, or spelt bread

- Parboil the lentils for 5 minutes and drain.
- Heat 1 Tbsp. oil in a 2-3 quart saucepan. Add the diced vegetables and cook over medium heat for several minutes, browning the lentils slightly.
- Add the crushed garlic and mash the tomato paste into the vegetables. Pour in the wine and stir in the mustard.
- Add 1 ½ cups water, the drained lentils, and 1 tsp. sea salt. Simmer, covered until the lentils are soft – 30-40 minutes. Wilt the spinach (or kale) over low heat in a skillet with the water clinging to its leaves.
- Season with sea salt and pepper (kale will take 7 minutes). Stir the cooked greens into the lentils. Add the oil, season to taste.
- Toast the bread and rub it with raw halved garlic. Cut each piece in thirds and arrange them on plates. Spoon the lentils over the toast and garnish with onions.

Desserts and Goodies

Grand Master Breakfast or Dessert Parfait

Here's a dessert that beautifies the skin, removes toxins, and helps get rid of those convoluted cottage cheese thighs.

- Yogurt fills your inner ecology with probiotics that help break down nutrients, encourage regularity and allow your skin to maximize the foods you consume.
- Bulk from the bran gleans away waste from the bowels and promotes bowel health.
- Bran aids in the removal of cholesterol from the blood. Excess circulating cholesterol can lead to bumpy, rough skin and clogged pores. Thus, controlling your cholesterol level can result in smoother skin.
- Apples deliver moisture and more fiber to colon which again supports regularity.
- Collectively, this dessert promotes beautiful skin by aiding in the efficient removal of toxins from the body while helping the skin retain an optimal moisture level.

1 half-cup of plain, organic yogurt-calcium (Look for organic Greek yogurt or coconut milk yogurt)
1 third-cup of all non-GMO bran cereal or granola
1 medium apple sliced into cubes
Blueberries, washed and dried
60% cacao nibs (cacao, not cocoa)
1 Tbsp. ground flax seeds

- In a tall glass add the cubed apples and top with the bran cereal. Top the cereal with the yogurt and repeat.
- As a dessert parfait, drizzle with Gran Marnier.
- Sprinkle on the cacao.
- Garnish with blueberries, flax, and walnuts.

Guiltless Chocolate Dipped Strawberries

Everyone feels happy and blissful while enjoying sweet, delicious and chocolate dipped strawberries, but sugar and cocoa butter create some health issues. Fret no more. Use this versatile dip for dipping all sorts of things or eat it by the spoonful in moderation. If you wish, maple syrup will sweeten this quite nicely.

Fresh, ripe strawberries, very cold
3 Tbsp. "cacao" powder (Notice the spelling)
3 Tbsp. raw, unrefined coconut oil
4-5 drops liquid Stevia or 2 portion control packages

- Wash and dry strawberries, leaving green stem on. Chill.
- Melt coconut oil and stir in cacao powder until smooth. It melts at 80° so no need to overheat it.
- Stir in Stevia. Cool.
- Dip chilled strawberries in to coat, setting on wax paper. Chill immediately.
- If you want to be naughty and have some fun, use a syringe and inject them in the center with Gran Mariner.

Orgasmic Vegan Chocolate Chip Cookies

Some of the best cookies I have ever tasted! Even my meat-eating family devoured these down. The cool part: limited ingredients and baking time is only 9 minutes!

2 cups organic unbleached flour
2 tsp. aluminum-free baking powder
1/2 tsp. Himalayan salt
1 tsp. cinnamon
3/4 cup vegan, dark chocolate, or cacao chips
3/4 cup raw coconut sugar
1/2 cup cold-pressed grape seed oil

1 tsp. vanilla extract
1/2 cup almond or coconut milk

- Preheat oven to 350°.
- In a large bowl, mix the flour, baking powder, salt, chocolate chips, and cinnamon.
- Make a "well" in the center of the dry ingredients and put aside.
- In a medium sized bowl, mix sugar, grape seed oil, vanilla extract, and milk replacement. Add more milk replacement for more cake-like texture.
- Pour wet ingredients into center of well in dry ingredients. Mix well, but do not overwork dough.
- Bake 350°, 5 minutes, rotate pan and bake 4 minutes, or until brown around the edges. Remove from oven and let cool.

Cacao Nib Trail Mix

This trail mix takes about 2 minutes to throw together. Perfect for cooks on the grab-and- go!

1 cup raw cacao nibs
1/2 cup raw walnuts
1/2 cup raw almonds
1 cup Goji berries
1 cup raw shredded coconut
Cinnamon to taste

- Combine all ingredients in a large bowl.
- Dust with cinnamon to taste, and store the trail mix in an airtight container or large zip-top bag.

Raw, Unprocessed Coconut Oil and Milk:

- Non hydrogenated
- A medium-chain saturated fat.
- Lauric, Caprylic, and Capric acid help maintain healthy cholesterol levels.
- Boosts the immune system.
- Natural anti-inflammatory healing properties.
- Effective treatment for Alzheimer's

- Improved IBS and Crohn's symptoms
- Rich in vitamins and minerals
- Antiviral, antimicrobial, antiprotozoal and antifungal. It kills all the bad stuff in your body.
- Boost energy and endurance
- Boosts thyroid function
- Improves insulin and blood glucose
- Protects against osteoporosis
- Protects against cancer
- Supports healing and skin repair.
- Softens skin, prevents wrinkles
- Conditions hair, controls dandruff
- Plus, you'll experience the best shave of your life

How to use it in the kitchen:
- Popcorn
- Smoothies
- Fry eggs
- Bake cookies and cakes
- Green Tea
- Sauté vegetables
- Over warm oatmeal with summer berries

Coconut Whipped Cream

1—15 ounce can of full-fat coconut milk (Refrigerate overnight)
1 tsp. vanilla extract
1 tsp. raw honey or
1 pkg. Stevia

- Without shaking it, open the can and spoon to layer of thickened coconut cream into a mixing bowl. Reserve milk or drink it.
- Whip coconut cream with electric beaters, starting on low and move to high until creamy. Move the beaters up and down to infuse cream with air.
- Add vanilla and sweetener. Stir and combine.
- Serve immediately or store in fridge for up to 3 days.

Chocolate Avocado Pudding

As counterintuitive as it sounds, this is totally delicious and wildly nutritious.

2 ripe avocados full of mono-unsaturated, antioxidant goodness
3 Tbsp. 100% pure maple syrup
¼ Cup organic blue agave syrup
1 ½ tsp. balsamic vinegar
2 tsp. vanilla extract
2/3 cup "cacao" powder
Pinch of Himalayan salt

- Put all ingredients into a blender or food processor and blend until creamy.
- Adjust flavor with a dash more balsamic.
- Refrigerate the leftovers if there are any.

Chocolate Banana Cream Coconut Pie

Crust:
1 1/2 cups nuts (try a combination of almonds and pecans)
1 1/2 cups dates
Salt and/or vanilla, if you want

Chocolate Cream:
2-3 avocados
1/3 cup organic, raw agave
Pinch salt
1/2 tsp. cinnamon
1/4 cup cocoa/cacao
2 Tbsp. mesquite (optional)
2 Tbsp. melted coconut oil

Whipped Cream:
- 1 can chilled, full fat coconut milk (for a 100% raw version you can blend young Thai coconut meat with coconut oil and let it set in the fridge until firm).
- 3 Tbsp. raw powdered sugar (coconut sugar ground in a food processor works well!).

- Seeds from ½ vanilla bean.

To make the crust:
- Pulse nuts in food processor until they're the size of crumbs
- Add dates and pulse until it lumps together. Feel free to add cinnamon, salt, vanilla or more sweetener here
- Press into your favorite pie pan and stick in the fridge.

To make the chocolate cream
- Blend/process all ingredients until silky smooth.
- Now slice 3-4 bananas and put them on the bottom of the crust.
- Spoon on the chocolate cream and put on another player of banana slices. Set in the fridge again.

Right before serving
- CAREFULLY take out coconut milk from the fridge. Spoon the thick fat from the top; you want this. (There was about 1/2 a can left of milk when I got all the thick stuff).
- Put the milk you spooned out into a mixing bowl (Kitchen Aid) with the sugar and beat until thick and fluffy!
- Spoon onto your pie and voila! Enjoy.

Recipe from the website: Raw Food Recipes

Apple Pie Energy Bar
Makes about 6-7 bars

3/4 cups dried apples
3/4 cups pitted dates (about 18)
1/2 cup raisins (sultanas)
1/2 cup raw walnuts
1 1/2 – 2 tsp. ground cinnamon

- In a food processor combine the apples, dates, raisins and cinnamon and blend for a couple of minutes until a ball is formed

- Add the walnuts and blend until the walnuts are chopped to desired size
- Press firmly onto a piece of parchment paper forming a large rectangle about 1/2 inch wide
- Cool in the refrigerator for a couple of hours.
- Cut into desired shape.
- Store in an airtight container in the refrigerator

Grilled Summer Peaches with Goats Cheese, Lavender, Hazelnuts and Honey

¼ cup fresh goat's cheese
4 ripe peaches, washed thoroughly
3 Tbsp. EVOO
Lavender pedals
Mint springs
Whole hazelnuts (chopped)

- Remove goat's cheese from wrapper, place it in a bowl and let get to room temperature to soften.
- Cut the peaches in half along the seam that runs round the juicy stone fruit.
- Remove the stone carefully.
- Heat a sauté pan over medium high heat and pour in olive oil.
- Place peach halves meat side down into the hot oil and cook for about 1 minute.
- Add a dash of water to the goat's cheese and stir until it's workable.
- Place a generous spoonful of goat's cheese in the indentation of each peach.
- Sprinkle on lavender pedals.
- Drizzle with honey.
- Garnish with fresh mint leaves and hazelnuts (Filberts).

Peanut Butter Chocolate Chip Cookie Dough Bites
Yields about 14 1 1/2″ cookie dough balls.

You won't believe they're flourless and contain no oil or sugar.
Don't even try with regular peanut butter made from margarine!
They'll come out oily. Use organic peanut butter.

1 1/4 cups canned or freshly boiled chickpeas, well-rinsed and
patted dry with a paper towel
2 tsp. vanilla extract
1/2 cup + 2 Tbsp. natural peanut butter
1/4 cup raw honey or raw organic agave
1 tsp. aluminum-free baking powder
1 Tbsp. chia seeds
Pinch sea salt if your peanut butter doesn't have salt in it
1/2 cup semi-sweet dark chocolate chips

- Preheat oven to 350°F/175°C.
- Combine all the ingredients, except the chocolate chips
  in a good processor and process until very smooth.
  Make sure to scrape the sides and top to get the little
  chunks of chickpeas and process again until they're
  combined.
- Add the chocolate chips and stir if you can, or pulse
  once or twice. The mixture will be very thick and sticky.
- With wet hands, form into 1 ½ inch balls. Place onto a
  piece of parchment paper lined cookie sheet. If you
  want them to look more like normal cookies, press
  down slightly on the top of the balls. They do not raise
  much during baking. Bake for about 10 minutes,
  rotating pan after 5 minutes.

Raw Summer Berry and Peach Crumble

The less you do to a food, the more it can do for you! Raw foods are getting lots of attention and the wildly healthy trend is becoming more popular.

Crumble Topping:
1 cup walnuts
1/2 cup pitted, packed dates
1/2 cup shredded coconut
1 Tbsp. ground flax seed
1/3 cup ground raw oats
1/2 tsp. pure vanilla extract
Pinch Himalayan salt
1-2 tsp. water

- In a food processor, grind all ingredients together into a crumbly, yet moist texture.
- If you want the mixture to press together a bit better, add 1-2 teaspoons of water.
- Transfer to a bowl and make the filling.

Filling:
2/3 cup blueberries and red raspberries, rinsed under cold water
3-4 dates pitted and chopped into small bits
1-2 tsp. lemon juice
1/2 cup diced juicy peach (washed and unpeeled)

- Blend / pulse the first seven topping ingredients in a food processor.
- Add water a bit at a time until desired consistency is achieved.
- Place the majority of the crumble into and 8 x 8 pan and press down to pack.
- Gently spoon in the berries and peaches evenly.
- Sprinkle the remaining crumble over the top.
- Garnish with mint sprigs, red and blue berries.

Coconut Crack Bars

1 cup shredded coconut (unsweetened)
1/4 cup raw agave or pure maple syrup (or 1/4 cup water and 2-3 stevia packs)
2 Tbsp. EVOO
1/2 tsp. real vanilla extract
1/8 tsp. Himalayan salt

- Combine all ingredients in a food processor. (Perhaps, you can mix by hand if you don't have a food processor, but I haven't tried).
- Squish into any small container (I used a 7x5) and refrigerate for an hour before trying to cut. You may freeze for 15 minutes. This may be stored in the fridge or freezer for a few weeks.

Simple Cha-Cha-Chia Pudding Pie

Base:
1 cup dates (remove two dates to reduce the sweetness)
1 cup pecans
¼ tsp. real vanilla
Pinch Himalayan salt

Pit and soak the dates for 5 minutes. Grind nuts into a flour in your blender or food processor. Add the rest of the ingredients and process until you have dough. Press down the dough on a plate or pie form measuring about 8 inches across.

Filling:
1 cup berries of your choice (save some for the topping)
3 tsp. of raw agave nectar or raw honey
2 Tbsp. of chia seeds
1/4 tsp. real vanilla
half a banana

- Add all of the filling ingredients to your blender. Pour the filling over the base and add some berries on top. Put in the fridge to chill a couple of hours or overnight.

Sugar-Free Oatmeal Raisin Cookies
Yield: 24-30 cut out cookies

1/2 cup brown rice syrup
1/3 cup vegan grape seed oil or vegan margarine
1 cup raisins
2 Tbsp. real vanilla
1/2 tsp. almond extract
1 cup of cooked steel cut oatmeal (avoid "Instant" versions)
2 Tbsp. ground flax seeds
1 1/2 cups gluten-free flour
1/2 cup arrowroot
1 tsp. aluminum-free baking powder
1/2 tsp. Himalayan salt
(Optional toppings: chopped dried fruits, and chopped nuts, etc.)

- Pre-heat oven to 350°
- Line a cookie sheet with parchment paper or non-stick baking liners and set aside. In a small bowl, place the brown rice syrup, oil, vanilla, and almond extract, and whisk well to combine.
- In a medium bowl, place the flour, arrowroot, baking powder, and salt, and stir well to combine.
- Add the raising and wet ingredients to the dry ingredients and stir until well blended.
- Gather the dough into a ball and divide in half. Work with one half of the dough at a time and cover the remainder to prevent it from drying out. Sprinkle a large piece of waxed paper with a little additional flour and place the dough on the floured waxed paper.
- In your squeaky-clean hands, gently form the cookies no more than ¼ inches thick.
- Place on the prepared cookie sheets.
- Bake at 350° for 8-10 minutes or until lightly browned on the bottom and around the edges.

Allow the cookies to cool on the cookie sheets for a few minutes before transferring them to a rack to cool completely. When all of the cookies are cooled completely, store them in an airtight container with waxed paper between the layers.

Chewy Chocolate Chunk Cookies

These are grain-free, refined sugar free and amazing! They are made with almond butter and raw honey.

Preheat oven to 350 degrees
1 cup of unsalted almond butter, or sun butter if you are nut-free
1/2 cup raw honey melted
2 Tbsp. coconut flour
1 egg
1/2 tsp. aluminum-free baking soda
1 pinch Himalayan salt
About 4 oz. (I used half of a bar) of 85% or higher dark chocolate. I like "Green and Black's" organic brand

- Mix all ingredients except for chocolate in a large bowl
- Chop the chocolate into chunks and fold it in
- using a cookie scooper, scoop onto parchment paper lined cookie sheet
- Bake for 10 minutes, rotating pan after 5 minutes
- Let them set for 20 minutes before eating.

Raw Carrot Cake
One 9" cake

Raw desserts are super refreshing, healthy, living sweets that are so easy to make as they require absolutely no cooking or baking, ideal for saving energy during the summer months.

For the crust:
2 cups finely ground raw almonds
½ tsp. Himalayan salt
½ cup finely chopped Medjool dates
1/3 cup maple syrup
½ cup raw sunflower seeds

For the Filling:
1 pound carrots, finely grated
1 16-ounce bag frozen pineapple, thawed
1/3 cup finely ground raw cashews

For the Frosting:
1 1/3 cups finely ground raw macadamia nuts
2 cups finely chopped Medjool dates
1/4 cup maple syrup
¼ cup fresh lemon juice

- Line the bottom of a 9" spring-form pan with parchment paper.
- **Make the crust**. In a food processor, blend the almonds, salt, dates, and maple syrup until creamy. Mix in the sunflower seeds and press into the prepared pan. Place the pan in the freezer for at least 30 minutes before adding the filling.
- **Make the filling**. In a food processor, blend the carrots, pineapple and cashews until just combined. Spread the mixture on top of the crust layer and place in the refrigerator for 15 minutes.
- **Make the frosting**. In a blender or food processor, blend the ground macadamia nuts, dates, lemon juice and maple syrup until creamy.
- Spread over the filling and chill in the refrigerator for 30 minutes before serving. Serve cold.

Raw Banana Nut Bars

For the crust:
1 cup finely ground rolled oats (from about 1 1/3 cup rolled oats)
1 cup finely ground raw almonds
1/2 cup finely chopped Medjool dates
1/2 tsp. Sea salt
1/4 cup agave nectar or maple syrup
2 Tbsp. Fresh orange juice, plus more if needed

For the Filling:
1 cup finely ground raw cashews
3 cups mashed ripe banana
1/2 cup finely chopped Medjool dates
2 Tbsp. maple syrup
2 Tbsp. raw, unrefined coconut oil
1/4 tsp. Himalayan salt
1/4 cup chopped walnuts (optional)

- Line an 8" x 8" pan with parchment and set aside. In a medium-sized mixing bowl, combine the finely ground rolled oats, ground almonds, Medjool dates and sea salt.
- Add the agave nectar and orange juice, mixing until the mixture just holds together but is not wet, adding more orange juice if necessary. Press half of the mixture into the bottom of the prepared pan and place in the freezer for about 1 hour.
- **Make the banana filling**. In a blender, process all of the ingredients except for the chopped walnuts until creamy. Stir in the chopped walnuts by hand, transfer to a mixing bowl, and place in the freezer for 30 minutes to an hour.
- Spread the banana mixture on top of the crust. Press the remaining crust mixture on top of the banana mixture. Return the pan to the freezer for 1 hour.
- Serve cold and enjoy!

Peanut Butter Bars
Makes 16 bars

1 cup organic peanut butter (hold the trans-fats, please)
1/ cup brown rice syrup or sorghum
3/4 cup chopped raw walnuts
1 tsp. cinnamon
1 1/2 tsp. vanilla extract
4 cups organic puffed or crisped brown rice cereal or any other puffed or crisped whole grain cereal like millet, spelt or quinoa
8 X 8 glass baking vessel

- Blend together the peanut butter, sweetener, cinnamon, and vanilla.
- Gently fold in the cereal and walnuts until combined.
- Press into a lightly oiled 8 X 8 glass pan and cover with waxed paper.
- Refrigerate for at least 1 hour before diving in.
- Store in the fridge if they last that long.

No-Bake Chocolate Oatmeal Cookies

2 cups organic sugar
1/2 cup plain almond milk
1/4 cup vegan margarine
3 Tbsp. Dutch cocoa
3 cups organic "quick" oats
1/2 cup organic peanut butter
1 tsp. vanilla extract

- In a saucepan cook sugar, soy milk, margarine and cocoa to hard rolling boil. Boil for 1 minute.
- Remove pan from stove, quickly add peanut butter, vanilla, and then the oats.
- Mix quickly and drop by the spoonful on wax paper.
- Add chopped walnuts if desired for the Omega 2 boost.

Beverages

Turmeric Tea

There's lots of news lately about the glorious healing and detoxing properties of the ancient spice, Turmeric. It a free-radical-fighting antioxidant hailed as defense against both cancer and Alzheimer's. Ginger is its BFF. In India, turmeric combined with fresh ginger is part of the daily diet with Alzheimer's rates four times less than in the U.S. Americans don't use it for the intended reasons; it was gifted to us by creation. We use turmeric to color mustard, cheddar cheese, clothing, pickles, and butter. Durkee and McCormick's brands are DOA, so get it from your community health store. In bulk it's cheaper.

Turmeric:

- Vacuums up free radical debris that can cause disease.
- Cools the fires of inflammation.
- Improves digestion.
- Cleanses the liver.
- People with the following conditions could benefit from it. IBS, colitis, Crohn's disease, diarrhea, and post-giardia or post salmonella conditions.
- Can reduce the itching and inflammation of hemorrhoids.
- Turmeric can affect those on Coumadin/Warfarin. Turmeric thins the blood so you will need to adjust your medications.

Ingredients:

- 2 cups filtered, boiling water
- 1 Inch fresh ginger, smashed (no need to peel)
- ½ tsp. powdered turmeric
- 1/8 tsp. cayenne
- ¼ cups Bragg's cider vinegar
- 1 Tbsp. raw local honey or local maple syrup (Stevia is okay too)
- ½ lemon, seeded

Made in the USA
Lexington, KY
08 August 2015